W9-BXY-406

Dedication

We dedicate this book to those
health-conscious consumers
who value their teeth and are looking
for caring, comprehensive dentistry.
If your dentist shared this book with you,
congratulate yourself — you have found
the right dentist.

Table of Contents

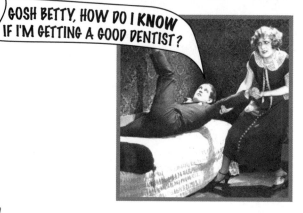

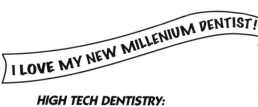

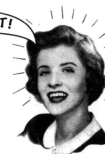

HIGH TECH DENTISTRY:
That Was Then, This Is Now:
Compare the 1930s dental office
to the office of the 21st century.

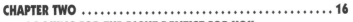

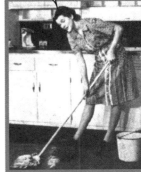

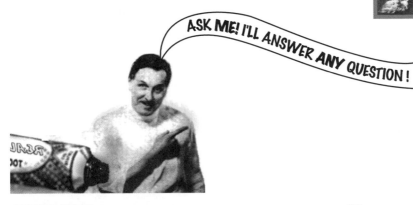

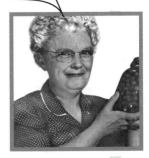

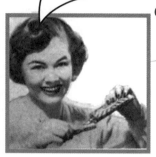

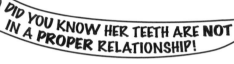
I JUST STENCIL THE KIDS' NAMES ON THEIR TOOTHBRUSHES.

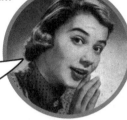
DID YOU KNOW HER TEETH ARE **NOT** IN A PROPER RELATIONSHIP!

SECTION III 61
YOUR MOUTH:
The Gateway to Your Health

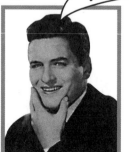
NOTHIN' PASSES THESE LIPS THAT CAN HURT MY HEART!

LOOK! THERE'S YOUR FIRST TOOTH!

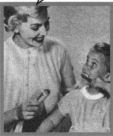

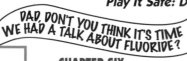

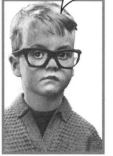

OH HENRY! I JUST TINGLE WHEN YOU TALK ROOT CANALS!

ONLY MY DENTIST KNOWS FOR SURE . . .

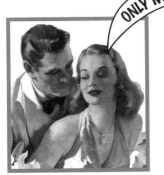

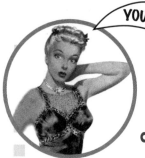

YOU MEAN I NEED TO IMPROVE MY SMILE!

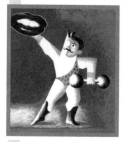

THE MINUTE I FINISH THIS SANDWICH I'LL PULL OUT MY FLOSS & TOOTHBRUSH.

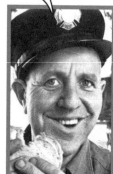

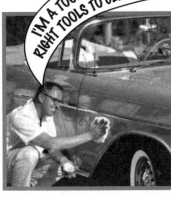

I'M A TOOL GUY ... I LIKE HAVING THE RIGHT TOOLS TO CLEAN MY TEETH TOO!

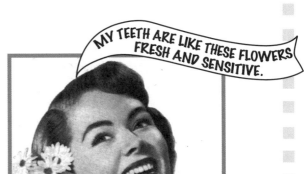

MY TEETH ARE LIKE THESE FLOWERS FRESH AND SENSITIVE.

Acknowledgments

*A*sk an artist how long it took to create a particular painting and he or she will often answer, "A lifetime." So it was with the creation of this book. By a funny quirk of fate, I bumped into Mac Lee and Joleen Jackson in a small town located in the Texas Hill Country, which was where we first discussed writing a consumer brochure. They wanted to reach dental consumers just like me to help them move beyond hating the dentist and into a place of health. Well, as you can see, that brochure grew into a sizable book. And before we launch into our many thanks, I would like to tip my hat to my co-authors for so generously sharing their vast experience and knowledge and for allowing me to transcribe their honesty and passion for dentistry onto the pages of this book.

The training and experience we have each gained from our individual professions make it impossible to acknowledge all of the people we should here. But first and foremost, we wish to express our love and thanks to our families for their continued support and encouragement, which was essential in a project of this magnitude. In addition, Mac Lee wishes to acknowledge his wife, Carol Ann Lee, for her belief and support in all his endeavors.

Many talented professionals have shared their dental knowledge and conveyed a standard of integrity that has left an enduring impression on Dr. Mac Lee and Joleen Jackson. These colleagues include: The L.D. Pankey Institute, Dr. Peter Dawson, and Dr. Earl Estep (who was an especially unselfish and encouraging mentor). We also want to thank our dedicated study group for their constant support and for sharing their professional experience and insights over the years. Included in this acknowledgement are Dr. Lee's loyal dental team members. They contribute so much each day to making his dental office a comfortable refuge that even patients who hate dentists love to visit.

Just as a dentist requires the assistance of an entire team of professionals to care for your dental health, so we drew on the friendship and special training of several talented dentists who shared their expertise with us. They deserve significant credit and kudos and include: pediatric dentist Gordon Strole; orthodontist Robert Westbrook, Jr.; and Dr. Robert (Buddy) Lee for the time he spent sharing his training and his achievements in cosmetic dentistry. We are especially grateful to Dr. Stan Shelton for sharing his extensive knowledge of dental technology and for the use of his high-tech equipment, which provided us with the digital images used in the book. We also wish to extend our appreciation and thanks to Dr. John Kois, an exceptional dentist and a master in clinical instruction, for his wise guidance and for providing us with examples of his work.

And finally, a big round of applause goes to our hardworking editorial, design, and technical support team. Jim Audette, for his fine writing contributions and editorial guidance; Gretchen Douma, for her keen editorial eye; Brandon Fickel, our computer guru and technology expert; and Morgan Brooke, who wore many design and illustration hats and looked good in all of them.

Last, but by no means least, Dr. Lee and Joleen Jackson wish to give their personal acknowledgment to all of the patients who over the years began their dental appointments by sharing how much they hated to be there and ended their visits in a trusting dental partnership.

Thanks to Y'all

Nothin' Personal Doc, But
I HATE DENTISTS!

I can't tell you how many times we've heard patients say this as they walk in the door. It's quite an irony— so many people love their teeth, but hate the dentist. But if you think about it, it's not hard to understand. We love our teeth because they are such a basic part of our sensory existence. We literally need them to live. By contrast, dentists are perceived as the people who use sharp instruments to poke, pry, and pull at our beloved teeth.

Of course, the logical problem with this reasoning is that avoiding the dentist is one of the surest ways to lose your beloved teeth.

That's why I have wanted to write this book for a long time. I believe that given the right information, health-conscious consumers will see their dentists in a totally different light—as an ally and an advocate for healthy teeth and gums. My goal is not to improve the image of dentistry but rather to empower consumers to get the best dental care possible.

To help write this consumer guide, I've enlisted some help from the "real" world. Joleen Jackson and I have trained thousands of dentists and dental team members over the past 15 years, so we understand the way they think and how they operate. Three years ago, Joleen expanded her training focus to include educating patients. Her work as a professional liaison and educator to new dental patients uncovered many of the consumer issues and concerns that we tackle in this book.

Vicki Audette has been a veteran consumer reporter for more than 20 years. She's made it her business to understand what consumers are looking for and how they expect to be treated. Besides collaborating on every aspect of this book, you'll find her "Critic's Corner" and her personal dental profile useful reality checks for the everyday dental consumer.

By chance, the three of us joined forces about four years ago as consultants to dentists who wanted to become better communicators in their practices. Working together, we quickly began to identify numerous ways of improving the relationship consumers have with their dentists. Our greatest hope is that we can arm you with insights about the health of your teeth and help you choose wisely dentistry that is right for you and your family.

Today dentistry is faster, easier, and far less painful than ever. And the range of consumer choices—from advanced dental technologies to the variety of options available for restoring teeth—is unprecedented. Overcoming the obstacles that may have kept you from getting essential dental work will be easier when you realize that you are a partner in the care of your teeth. Good dentists will be excited about your new attitude and your informed questions. The rest may be intimidated. You'll be able to tell the difference.

As a dentist, I understood very early that having a sense of humor was an important ingredient for building a trusting relationship with my patients. We have tried to make your reading fun, as well as informational. You can tell from the title of this book that it was never meant to be a dental textbook, and every page was written with your best interest in mind. So here's to loving your teeth for the rest of your life and loving your dentist.

Dr. McHenry "Mac" Lee

SECTION I:

IT'S AN OLD STORY:
Dental Fear and Loathing

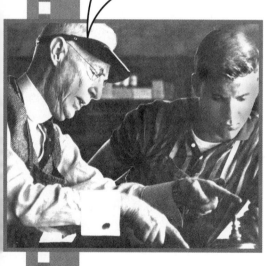

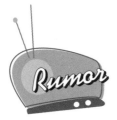

Rumor

Years ago, whenever I went to the dentist it really hurt. I was so miserable that I haven't been back.

Today dentistry and advanced technology have successfully merged and dramatically changed the experience of going to the dentist. Modern comforts and high-tech equipment offer patients almost painless dental visits.

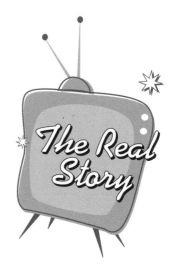

The Real Story

Why people hate dentists

Section Highlights

- ◆ Overcome dental fear and anxiety
- ◆ New comforts and pain relief
- ◆ High-tech dentistry
- ◆ Find the right dentist
- ◆ Money and insurance

During the 1950s, TV was coming of age with shows like *Howdy Doody, Sky King, Hopalong Cassidy,* and *The Honeymooners.* The "tube" entered households at the speed of Superman and became a national pastime. Also popular were fallout shelters, poodle skirts, and duck tail haircuts. What wasn't popular, however, was going to the dentist, but that's no surprise. For hundreds of years, dentists have been a ripe source of frightening imagery for artists. And many baby boomers grew up dreading the smell of the dental office and the noise and vibration of the "dreaded" slow drill of that time.

The dental office of the year 2000 bears no resemblance to what it was in the 1930s, '40s, or '50s and the old jokes no longer suit the technically sophisticated profession that dentistry is today. As a result, many folks who haven't been to the dentist for awhile are not aware how far dentists, dental labs, and manufacturers have traveled to give patients the highest level of comfort.

In this section, we deal with your fears and anxieties and any issues of mistrust that can keep you from going to the dentist. We arm you with information and questions to ask when searching for the right dentist for you. We also take you backward and forward in time. In "That Was Then, This Is Now," we will show you how technology has skyrocketed dentistry into the new millennium. So sit back and relax. This won't hurt a bit.

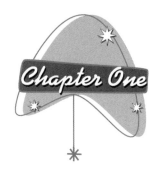

KEEP YOUR TEETH ALIVE!
Put a Modern Spin on an Old Dental Story

Chapter One

*W*hen we first started writing this book, it seemed as if the number one problem for people who say, "Nothin' personal doc, but I hate dentists!" is the fear and anxiety created by the nightmarish dental experiences of childhood. In some cases, the experiences were difficult. But, after much heated debate, we concluded that the core issue is a lack of trust because folks don't understand what the dentist is doing to their teeth and gums. And lack of trust can create feelings of fear and anxiety, shame and embarrassment, and claustrophobia.

To keep your teeth alive, we are determined to help you leap over tall buildings and overcome smile-defeating obstacles that keep you from getting your teeth fixed or put you into a cold sweat every time you walk into a dental office. The fact is, however, that most of us want to keep our teeth and the only person who can help us do that is a dentist. And one thing we know for certain, when people get their teeth and gums into a healthy prevention mode and work on a daily mouth care regimen, a trip to the dentist is a walk in the park.

When you buy a new car and bring it in for the recommended warranty check-ups, it makes you feel secure that no unexpected problems are going to occur—unless of course you get into an accident. It's somewhat similar with teeth. When you get your teeth up to speed and functioning in optimal health, you'll get a lot more mileage on your teeth—for less money—than you will on that new car.

Say It Loud, Say It Clear

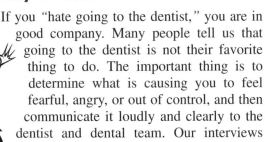

If you "hate going to the dentist," you are in good company. Many people tell us that going to the dentist is not their favorite thing to do. The important thing is to determine what is causing you to feel fearful, angry, or out of control, and then communicate it loudly and clearly to the dentist and dental team. Our interviews revealed that people who hate dentists can have a greatly enhanced and positive experience in a dental office:

- ◆ If they trust their dentist and dental team.
- ◆ If they have full confidence that they will be in total control.
- ◆ If they know exactly what to expect during the dental procedure.
- ◆ If they are confident that they will be numb or can be sedated in some way.

What follows are dental stories that demonstrate the type of concerns patients commonly express.

A Story of Fear and Anxiety

Darn! I got a headache or something. I'll cancel Dr. McLee again.

"The dentist said I was numb and I wouldn't feel anything. But I wasn't numb and when I told him, he didn't believe me. He dismissed me, and at that point, I lost my faith and trust in dentists."

People can develop strong fear and anxiety around going to the dentist when they hear dental "horror" stories from friends or co-workers. Or they become distrustful, especially if they've had a bad dental experience like the "I wasn't numb" story we just related. In some cases, they never get past their fears long enough to make another dental appointment. We've even heard some women say, *"I'd rather go through labor than go to the dentist."*

The Real Story

It's necessary to develop a rapport with your dentist and dental team. This is crucial because not only is fear a problem, but trust is an issue too. If you are very apprehensive, you will need to search for the dental professionals who are willing to take the time to reassure and support you. There are dental offices that pride themselves in caring for "high fear" patients. Everyone deserves a caring dental team who will discuss the variety of comfort and pain-relieving options available. The dentist can also assure you that you will be in control and listened to every step of the way. If you say that you are feeling pain or holler stop, be assured that all work will stop.

A Story of Distrust

My whole soy bean crop is goin' into the wife's teeth!

"I paid a lot of money for a root canal and the #@!% thing didn't work and I had to have the tooth pulled anyway."*

"They told me my son had 10 cavities and he was just to the dentist six months ago."

"The dentist said my tooth was cracked and I needed a crown, and that tooth never did hurt me."

"Every time I go to the dentist, it seems that I have something wrong. What's he trying to do, put his kid through college?"

The list goes on and on. People with unpleasant dental experiences or those who have heard the horror stories of the past will naturally mistrust dentists. Their perception is: dentists have no sense of humor; they play golf all the time; they cause pain; they make a lot of money on "my" teeth; and they go on vacation every month and call it a seminar.

Since only the dentist has been to dental school, you have to trust what he or she is telling you and you really don't know what questions to ask. So your only answers are "Yes, let's do it" or "I'll think about it," which means "no" or that you don't believe the diagnosis.

The Real Story

Our best advice for you is to read the rest of this book to become an enlightened dental consumer. Next, find a dentist who welcomes open communication with a patient. When you feel deep in your heart that the dentist is listening and concerned about you and your dental needs, you have found the right dentist. Building a professional relationship that revolves around mutual respect and trust goes a long way in changing your negative feelings and perceptions.

A Story of Shame and Embarrassment

I traded a moment of dental neglect for a lifetime of shame!

"I'm so embarrassed. It has been several years since I've been to the dentist. You are just going to die when you see my teeth."

We all fear being embarrassed or being reproached for personal neglect. Some folks will avoid going to the dentist because they are afraid of being reprimanded for not taking care of their teeth. Fear of embarrassment causes procrastination. It becomes a vicious cycle. The longer you wait to go to the dentist, the faster the weeks turn into months and the months into years. The feelings of shame grow bigger and bigger as time slips quickly by. Eventually, a dental emergency arises and you are forced to get help somewhere.

The Real Story

You need to know that you are not alone. Dentists and hygienists treat patients who feel exactly as you do every day. Most dentists today are empathetic about patients in this situation. They know that people don't like going to the dentist and they know that they have to do their very best to make you feel comfortable. Making a patient feel guilty is off limits in a modern dental office. Your first visit is the first day of your new dental health commitment. You are to be congratulated for showing up, not reprimanded for waiting so long.

A Story of Claustrophobia

Floyd, I just need some space.

"I started to panic, but I didn't know what to do. It seemed like it took them forever to stop. I had to ask them twice."

Maybe you have never experienced a feeling of claustrophobia, but some people do when they go to the dental office. They experience a feeling of helplessness because they can't move around and they feel forced to lie in the same position. As an exercise in empathy, imagine for a second that one to two people have their hands and instruments in your mouth and they are peering and staring with deep intensity at something. You have no clue what they might be thinking—but you feel it's all about you. What the dentist and team members are thinking about is the tooth (or teeth) and the very precise style of work that they are performing. Trust us. It's not about you.

The Real Story

The mouth is an intimate, personal area, and some people get scared of not having control while lying down in the dental chair. Each of us has a personal space zone. When that zone is violated, it makes us nervous and uncomfortable. Dentists know they are in close proximity and literally "in your face." Unless you trust your dentist and dental team, getting your dental work done may seem like a major violation of your personal space. The right dentist will respect your concerns. But the only way the dentist can do that is if you communicate what you are feeling *before* any work gets started.

The most important thing you need to know is that you are in control. Always express your feelings to the dentist and/or any dental team member. Arrange for a signal to indicate that you want to stop a procedure or take a break. Raising your hand works well for this. When the dental team understands and listens to you, the problem goes away. If you feel that you are being dismissed or not listened to, *you* should probably go away.

Get Comfortable

Today modern pain control procedures will take care of more than 90% of the people who previously could not get numb during a dental procedure. Unfortunately, many of those folks haven't been back to the dentist for years and don't realize the changes and benefits of the new technology.

Pain is real and anxiety is real, but they come from different places. If either of them are obstacles to getting your dental work done, read on.

Anxiety is a different issue than pain. Anxiety must be dealt with according to the individual and his/her level of anxiety. For some people, reassurance and just knowing that they are in control and that they can trust the dental team is enough. For others, distraction during a dental procedure is all they need.

Distractions

✔ Using virtual reality glasses that will put you a million miles away from the dental office.

✔ Watching TV while getting a procedure done.

✔ Listening to your favorite music, watching a movie, or playing a video game.

You will find that some dental offices bake bread or light aromatherapy candles to stifle the "smell of the dental office," or they use automatic aroma dispensers and air filters. Special pampering may include warm, scented towels after treatments, heating pads, comforting blankets, or even a teddy bear.

BE AN INFORMED DENTAL CONSUMER

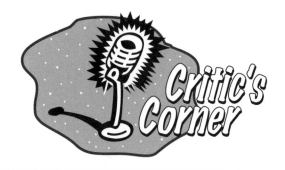

*W*ere you one of the millions of Americans a few years ago who read the *Reader's Digest* article, "How Honest Are Dentists?"

If you read it, you know that an investigative reporter traveled to 28 states and got 50 dental exams from 50 different dentists. He received a variety of diagnoses and was quoted a variety of treatment prices. At the close of the article, the reporter raised a valid question—how could all these dentists draw such different diagnoses from the same set of facts?

Many dentists were understandably upset. They were portrayed in the article as money-hungry opportunists. As readers, we were left feeling helpless—dental victims who could do nothing to avoid getting ripped off by a dentist.

To complicate matters, as consumers we know very little about our mouths and even less about what the dentist does to them. The truism *the more you know, the better you can make an informed decision* is as valid when shopping for dentistry as it is when shopping for a boat, a car, or furniture for your home.

Our mission is to help you become an interactive, educated partner in your dental care. We believe that by doing so, honesty and trust will just naturally follow.

Why Is There a Different Diagnosis from One Dentist to the Next?

1) Time

If you did not get a comprehensive exam, only some of your dental problems were diagnosed. The doctor must take the time to do a comprehensive exam. After that, there should be no surprises.

2) Training

A dentist is a dentist is a dentist. Right? Wrong! Technical skills will vary from one dentist to the next. Training doesn't end on the day the dentist graduates from dental school. It extends for as long as he or she practices dentistry.

3) Experience

With experience comes confidence. A dentist may be too scared to diagnose a patient's problem because he or she is not trained to fix it. (Or too scared to tell the patient the bad news). The dentist can have all the additional training available. But unless he or she has repeatedly *performed* the dental procedure in question, the dentist cannot predict the outcome. With experience and knowledge, the dentist will know whether or not a procedure will work because he or she has seen the results over and over again.

4) Integrity

A good dentist recommends treatment based on what is best for the patient—not what treatment will line his or her pockets with money. Sadly, greed rears its ugly head in all professions.

There Is Help for Your Anxiety

When it comes to using any kind of conscious or unconscious sedation including nitrous oxide, there are questions you need to ask beforehand. There are guidelines and protocols set by the American Dental Association (ADA) for both conscious and unconscious sedation. We recommend that you ask if your dental professional is following the ADA guidelines. Also ask, "Is this a procedure that you do in your office on a frequent basis?"

CONSCIOUS SEDATION (in-office procedures)

◆ Nitrous Oxide with Oxygen

Nitrous oxide, commonly called laughing gas, produces a mild level of conscious sedation that is helpful in decreasing anxiety. There are many advantages for using nitrous oxide. It is reversible almost immediately. In other words, the effect lasts only as long as the gas is being inhaled. And, if you don't like how it feels, the gas can be turned off at any time during a procedure.

◆ Oral Sedation

For adults who need a deeper state of sedation because their anxiety is very high, oral sedation is often used. Oral sedation is not as flexible as nitrous oxide because once the pill (or pills) is swallowed, you have to wait for the effects to wear off as the body eliminates the medication.

◆ Intravenous Sedation

For adults, intravenous sedation is used mostly in oral surgeons' and periodontists' offices where long, complicated surgical procedures are performed.

UNCONSCIOUS SEDATION

◆ General Anesthesia

General anesthesia is necessary for extremely complicated dental cases such as jaw surgery and/or for mentally or physically challenged individuals. We recommend that general anesthesia be done in the hospital where there is a full emergency staff available in case there are any problems.

Please Handle Me with Care

Put a check mark in the box next to the statement that concerns you or describes your problem. Then share this information with your dental team.

- [ ] I gag easily.
- [ ] I feel out of control when I'm lying down in the dental chair.
- [ ] I have not been to the dentist for a long time, and I feel uncomfortable about what you will say about my teeth and my dental hygiene.
- [ ] Pain relief is a top priority for me.
- [ ] I don't like shots (or I've had a bad reaction to shots).
- [ ] Please tell me what I need to know about my mouth in order to make an informed decision.
- [ ] My teeth are very sensitive.
- [ ] I don't like the sound of that tool that makes the picking and scraping noise. It's like someone is scratching fingernails on a blackboard.
- [ ] I don't like cotton in my mouth.
- [ ] I hate the noise of the drill.
- [ ] Please respect my time. I don't want to be left sitting in the reception area.
- [ ] I want to know the cost up front. No money surprises please.
- [ ] I have difficulty listening and remembering what I hear while sitting in the dental chair.
- [ ] I have health problems and questions that we need to discuss.

A *"Handle Me with Care"* Partnership

Now that you understand the importance of communicating all your fears and any issues of embarrassment and trust, let's look at making a "handle me with care" pact between you and your dental professionals. This simple, straightforward statement will make a big difference in how you are treated and how you feel about going to the dentist.

THE HANDLE ME WITH CARE PARTNERSHIP PACT:

I ask that you honestly inform me of all my dental problems. I want you to make me aware of the best quality dentistry available today. Then we can discuss how I can make healthy choices that will work within my budget. I also want to know all the pain relief options available to me in your dental office, how each dental procedure will work, and how much of my time will be required.

That Was Then...

Author Mac Lee is a third-generation dentist. His grandfather, Robert E. Lee, was a dentist, his father was a dentist, and his brother, Buddy Lee, is also a dentist. We decided to take advantage of all that history and do an inventory of Dr. Lee, Sr.'s dental office to see what it provided his patients during the 1930s compared to dental offices today. We found a huge difference. But you can read it for yourself.

The Dental Office of the '30s
For Fillings, Extractions, and Hygiene... Do You Remember?

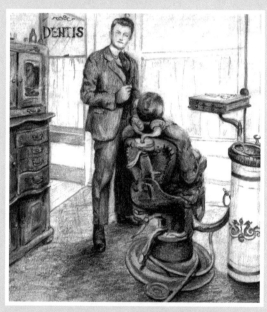

Author Dr. Mac Lee's grandfather's dental office, circa 1930. (drawing by Brenda Little)

✛ Slow speed drills
✛ Stand-up dentistry
✛ No way to eliminate dust made by the drill
✛ Spittoon
✛ Boil and re-use dental instruments for infection control
✛ Amalgam filling material squeezed into the dentist's hand
✛ No plastic fillings
✛ No radiation control on x-rays
✛ Hammer and chisel extractions
✛ Only novocaine to manage pain
✛ Blindfold for added comfort
✛ No insurance
✛ Limited infection control

...This Is Now!

COMFORTS & DISTRACTIONS

☑ Scented towels to clean yourself with after the dental procedure.

☑ Sit-down dentistry. Patient chairs recline and doctor sits.

☑ Buckwheat pillows.

☑ Fuzzy blankets.

☑ TV or movies at dental chair.

☑ Video games or music.

FILLINGS

- ☑ Air abrasion—A cavity prep that is less invasive than the high-speed drill.
- ☑ Tooth-colored fillings—Natural-looking and strengthens tooth structure.

DENTAL INSTRUMENTS

- ☑ High-speed handpiece—Replaces the old drill.
- ☑ Smaller, more precise instruments
- ☑ Laser drill—Has no vibration or high-pitched whine.
- ☑ Ultrasonic cleaning instruments

CROWNS & COSMETIC MATERIALS

- ☑ All-porcelain crowns
- ☑ Porcelain inlays
- ☑ Laser to shape gums
- ☑ Dental implants
- ☑ Fiber optic lights
- ☑ Teeth bleaching kits
- ☑ Laser bleaching
- ☑ Education videos for patients

ODOR CONTROL

- ☑ Aromatherapy
- ☑ Baking bread
- ☑ Flowers
- ☑ Automatic aroma dispensers

PAIN RELIEF

- ☑ Numbing gels
- ☑ Anti-anxiety medication
- ☑ Local anesthetics
- ☑ Conscious sedation (nitrous oxide with oxygen)
- ☑ Oral sedation

MAGNIFICATION TECHNOLOGY

- ☑ Ultra-magnified glasses for the dentist
- ☑ Intra-oral camera—A pencil-size wand outfitted with a camera to take pictures anywhere in the patient's mouth. The patient can see what the doctor is diagnosing.
- ☑ Digital imaging—Computerized color images (x-ray) show patients their teeth with 90% less radiation.

OFFICE MANAGEMENT

- ☑ Colorful uniforms
- ☑ Dental insurance
- ☑ Computers
- ☑ Electronic claims
- ☑ Phone head sets
- ☑ Patient education brochures

The list grows daily!

High-tech Cosmetic Restoration Dentistry

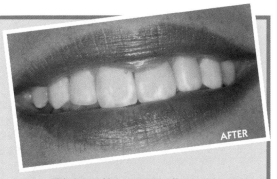

AFTER

This beautiful natural smile could never have been achieved without the new cosmetic technology.

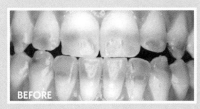

BEFORE

Tetracycline stained teeth

Chapter Two

LOOKING FOR THE RIGHT DENTIST FOR YOU

*O*vercoming the fear and mistrust of going to the dentist requires finding the right person to take care of your teeth and gums. But before we can advise you on how to find that person, you need to do a little soul-searching because dentistry is a product as well as a service. And, because it is also a highly *personalized* service, it is tough to write a list of hard and fast rules concerning how to find a dentist who is going to be just right for you. This is a process that will take you time, research, and interviewing.

What we can tell you for certain is that dedicated dentists take a sincere interest in their patients. And a good dentist and dental team respectfully treat the whole person, as well as the mouth. Your dental team will ask a lot of questions about your medical history and previous dental experience and, in turn, will eagerly answer your questions and concerns. Preventive dental care is their number one priority.

First Things First: Define *Your* Dental Priorities

Before you begin your search for Dr. Right, decide how healthy you want your mouth to be. Ask yourself two defining questions:

1. Are you serious about keeping your teeth for the rest of your life?

2. Do you only go to the dentist when you have a problem with a tooth or a dental emergency?

If you answered yes to the second question, almost any dentist can do the job you want. On the other hand, a resounding yes to the first question says that you are looking for a capable, prevention-minded dentist who will care for your dental health and help you hang on to one of your most cherished possessions—your teeth. In other words, you are looking for Dr. Right. Now that you've defined your dental priorities, you are ready for the next step—the search.

Looking for Dr. Right

There's more than one source for finding a Dr. Right. You can turn to the Yellow Pages, call a toll free referral service, read newspaper and magazine ads, find a name on a Web site, get a referral from a friend (or your former dentist), or select a name from a list provided by your dental insurance plan. It all boils down to making sure for yourself whether you are in the right place. Do your research and follow your instincts.

If you are looking for a new dentist and get a name from a friend, follow up with an interview phone call to the dental office. But don't stop there. Interview two or three additional dental offices. Ask questions and use our list of guidelines to help you determine professional and technical compatibility. One of the most important things to bring with you on your search is your intuitive powers. Yes, your intuition goes a long way in detecting whether the people you meet are sincere and whether you will be comfortable in their care.

In most cases, the phone will serve as your primary search tool. You can judge a lot about a dental practice from your first phone call. If the person answering the phone (the receptionist, front desk person, office manager or, heaven forbid, the dentist) is cheerful, helpful, patient, and answers all your questions, that is a good start and a signal that you may want to take it one step further. Ask about the office policy concerning new patients:

✔ Do they arrange a "get acquainted" visit with the dentist?

✔ Do they suggest a "walk through" of the office and an introduction to the dental team members?

✔ Do they have a designated staff person who routinely meets new patients and answers questions concerning the dental practice and its policies and procedures?

✔ Is it necessary to make an "on the books" dental appointment for a comprehensive dental examination?

Sink Your Teeth into This: Not every dental practice is set up to do "get acquainted visits" with the dentist, and very few have a designated staff member who handles new patient interviews. However, that is no indication of good or bad dentistry, and you shouldn't let it rule out a good prospect. In most cases, the standard operating procedure will be to schedule a first appointment with a dental examination. When this is the case, you want to make sure that you will get a comprehensive dental exam.

And remember, not every phone call is going to get you somewhere. Depending on who you call and where you live, you may feel that you are being brushed off, or you may sense that the person answering the phone is too rushed to answer your questions. It's also possible that you won't be able to get an appointment with the dentist for a couple of months. There are several reasons why this happens:

♦ The dental practice may be so good that there is a waiting list of people who want to become patients.

♦ Time management and appointment scheduling may be inefficient.

♦ The dental practice may have a "get them in and get them out" philosophy, which explains why you felt rushed.

♦ The person answering the phone may not be properly trained in customer service skills.

It's All about Choices and Communication

If you are not satisfied during the first part of your search—the phone call to the dental office—move on. If you are not satisfied with the second step—your initial dental visit and exam (or "get acquainted" visit)—move on. If you are not happy with the third step—the dentistry itself—it is time to express your feelings in person to the doctor. In other words, take charge. Let your fingers do the research, your mouth do the talking, and, by all means, vote with your feet.

It only makes sense to select your new dental home *before* any dental emergency arises. Nothing is more stressful than dealing with a toothache *and* severe pain *and* trying to locate Dr. Right at the same time. If you presently do not have a dentist, please leap into action.

Here are a few guidelines to follow and questions to ask when you are looking for the right dental professionals for you and/or your family:

☑ **Basic training:** A basic question—Does the dentist have a dental license? You can ask to see the license if you feel that is necessary. Since it is very difficult for you to judge the technical quality of the dentistry that's being done in your mouth, also inquire about the dentist's continuing education.

WHAT IS A GENERAL DENTIST?

The Academy of General Dentists (AGD) defines a general dentist as the primary care provider for patients in all age groups—a dentist who takes responsibility for the diagnosis, treatment, management, and overall coordination of services in order to meet the patient's oral health needs. To become a member of the AGD, a dentist must earn and document 75 hours of continuing dental education every three years (five years for recent dental school graduates). If a member dentist has a fellowship award (FAGD) (and roughly only 10% of all general dentists do), it means the dentist has completed 500 credit hours of continuing education and passed the Academy's Fellowship examination. The next step is an Academy Master (MAGD). A dentist must be a fellow first and then must have 600 additional hours of education. Four hundred of those 600 hours are hands-on training. By the time dentists have their fellowship and mastership, they have a minimum of 1100 hours of education. They must also meet yearly requirements to keep current.

☑ **Friendly, concerned service:** Are the dentist and team members friendly? Are they genuinely interested in you and committed to taking the time it takes to get to know you, to discuss your concerns, your fears, and your dental expectations? If you are a new patient, the dentist should give you a comprehensive exam and design a treatment plan that is appropriate for you based on your exam. Avoid a dental practice where the dentist and staff seem rushed, nervous, and unable to communicate with you.

☑ **Good information and listening skills:** Does the dentist involve you in discussing your treatment choices and options, rather than just telling you what to do? Does the dentist explain why the treatment is necessary, the benefits and drawbacks of the treatment, the possible risks, other repair or restoration options, and the cost?

When you are making treatment decisions, it's important for you to thoroughly discuss your dental priorities with your dentist. The following three questions are good ways to start a candid discussion:

1. Is this the treatment you would recommend for your family members?

2. How much time will this treatment require?

3. What will happen if I don't go ahead with the treatment?

Dr. Right will be happy to answer all your questions. In addition to the questions noted above, you can also ask:

☑ **Does the dentist wear special magnification lenses?** This is essential for doing quality work because dental procedures are precise and the dentist is working in a small, dark area on a small object. Most up-to-date dentists will tell you that they would not want to get their dental work done by a dentist who is not using high-tech, high-powered lenses.

☑ **Does the dentist or hygienist use a probing tool to check for gum disease when you have your teeth cleaned?** Avoid a dental office that does not routinely examine and discuss the health of your gums. If a gum evaluation using a probe has not been done, you need to find another dentist.

☑ **Does the dentist or hygienist use standard infection control procedures?** While experts agree that the chance of transmitting infectious diseases during routine visits to a dental office is remote, you will feel reassured if you know that the dentist is following OSHA and the ADA infection control guidelines. This means the dental team members wear gloves and masks, and all non-disposable instruments are heat and steam sterilized in an autoclave. Ask a team member what the dental office does for infection control. You can also ask to see the infection control area.

☑ **Look at the dentist's and the team members' teeth.** If they don't have healthy, good-looking smiles, maybe they haven't practiced good dentistry care themselves. If they aren't practicing good care, how can you be sure that they will be compassionate about your dental situation?

The Comprehensive Dental Exam

This all-important exam launches a lifelong master plan for your dental treatment—similar to an architect's blueprint. It is a thorough diagnosing tool and your appointment may take as long as an hour and a half. During that time, the doctor and the dental team are listening to your concerns and gathering facts about your medical history, which will be reviewed by the dentist before the exam begins. This examination records the "big picture" of your dental health. It is a diagnosing and planning appointment that every dental patient should experience.

Sink Your Teeth into This: The comprehensive dental exam is an honest plan that lets you know about all the disease in your mouth and forecasts what dental work will be necessary. It represents a standard of care in dentistry and provides the patient with a yardstick to measure the integrity of the dentist. Periodically the exam is updated to confirm the state of your dental health.

What to Expect During the Comprehensive Dental Exam

The dentist will be looking for decay, bone loss, abscesses, missing teeth, cancer, tumors, extra teeth, wisdom teeth, and any other mouth abnormalities. This thorough exam will give the dentist all the necessary information to make a complete diagnosis.

The exam should include:

◆ A medical history

◆ An oral cancer examination

◆ A periodontal evaluation to check for gum and bone disease

◆ Individual teeth checked visually for decay

◆ Bite checked to see if teeth fit together properly

◆ 18 x-rays or digital images (less if you do not have all of your teeth) to check for decay and bone loss and any other abnormalities

◆ Panoramic x-ray and/or models of the teeth, if necessary

MY LAST DENTIST DIDN'T TAKE THIS MANY X-RAYS

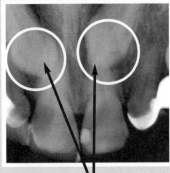

Why so many x-rays? Here's a good example of why the dentist must take x-rays of every tooth. This person was surprised to discover that two permanent teeth were hiding for 30 years! Now the patient knows they exist and the dentist can monitor the teeth for abscesses.

DENTISTS WHO PAY THEIR DUES

Dentists may belong to a variety of associations and organizations. These groups can range from being fee-based or training-based organizations to those groups whose members are admitted because of their achievement of specific clinical skills or by invitation because of their status within the dental community. Becoming a member of an association or organization and taking continuing education courses is only one way to measure whether a dentist is a good dentist. Paying dues to belong to an organization does not mean that every dentist who is a member will have the same level of training or technical skills. Ask your dentist if he or she belongs to any associations or organizations and ask about his/her continuing education. Your dentist will enjoy the opportunity to tell you about him or herself, and you will get an opportunity to judge his/her level of dedication to the profession.

18 DIGITAL IMAGES TAKEN DURING A COMPREHENSIVE DENTAL EXAM

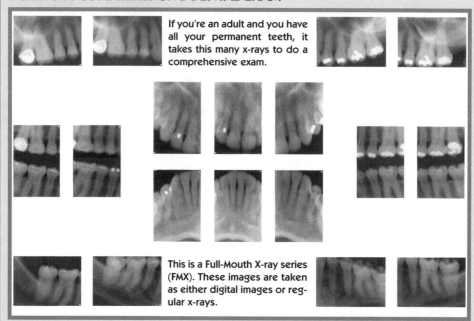

If you're an adult and you have all your permanent teeth, it takes this many x-rays to do a comprehensive exam.

This is a Full-Mouth X-ray series (FMX). These images are taken as either digital images or regular x-rays.

Benefits of the Comprehensive Exam

◆ **AVOID FUTURE TROUBLE:** A comprehensive examination creates a baseline of your overall dental health. If there is any change or progression of disease, the dentist can monitor it.

◆ **NO UNNECESSARY SURPRISES:** Your dentist will present you with a lifelong dental health plan to meet both your immediate needs and your future needs. Together, you and the dentist can discuss what dental options and opportunities are available to you in order to maintain optimal health. Major problems can be avoided or minimized (except, of course, for emergencies such as a broken tooth or toothache).

◆ **SCHEDULE YOUR TIME:** From start to finish, you will know how much dental work you need and how much time will be involved. You have an opportunity to schedule dental appointments to suit your needs.

◆ **PLAN YOUR BUDGET:** Avoid any guesswork. The financial coordinator at your dental clinic will give you the cost estimates of your dental repairs and restorations, so you can ask questions about your dental insurance benefits and make financial decisions that fit the dental costs into your budget.

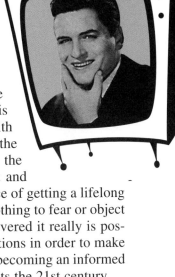

I was wrong! Things **are** different now.

Time for a New Attitude!

Have you noticed that the old dental story is really taking on a new twist as you come to the end of Chapter Two? Those who say "I hate the dentist" have many objections including "the dentist is always finding something new wrong with my teeth." But a person who can find the right dentist, who knows what to say to the dental team in order to develop rapport and trust, and who understands the importance of getting a lifelong master plan for good dental health has nothing to fear or object to. We hope by now that you have discovered it really is possible to overcome dental fears and objections in order to make healthy choices for your mouth. You are becoming an informed dental consumer with an attitude that suits the 21st century.

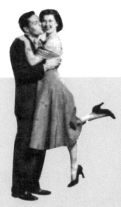

IT TAKES TWO TO TANGO

Since it takes two to tango, a good relationship between you and your dentist takes communication and effort. Here are a few dos and don'ts that will put you on the most valuable patient list:

✔ Do listen carefully to your dental diagnosis and treatment options.

✔ Don't be afraid to ask "silly" questions. If you are feeling anxious, you can't always listen effectively. So, if you don't understand what is being explained to you, ask the dentist or staff to clarify or write down the information.

✔ Don't dictate your treatment before you have been informed of all your options. ("Just pull the tooth, doc," or "Just patch that tooth up again.")

✔ Do you know how you digest information? For example, are you a "just the facts" type of person? Or do you want to know all the technical details? Let the dental team know *how* to communicate with you and everyone will be more comfortable.

A QUESTION OF INSURANCE AND MONEY

Dental insurance can be a "good thing," as Martha Stewart would say. Thanks to dental insurance, millions of adults and children use their benefits to visit a dental office on a regular basis. And it's been dental insurance that has brought volumes of people to dental offices for those all-important teeth cleanings.

Dental insurance has long been a mosaic of contradictions. It's a benefit for which there has never been a clear consensus on who pays what—or how much—among dentists, consumers, and insurance companies. Many people share a common misconception that dental insurance will pay 100% of their dental work. But every insurance company is different—what each insurance company pays is a percentage of what they consider "usual and customary."

The reactions of surprise and the disappointment people feel about dental insurance may be partly due to semantics. For most of us, the word "insurance" carries certain expectations. If, for example, we are in a car accident we expect our insurance to cover the repair costs of our car. If we require heart bypass surgery, we expect our insurance to pay a certain portion of the hospitalization and surgery. We understand auto and medical insurance policies and only occasionally do we encounter an unexpected surprise. Not so with dental insurance.

YOUR POLICY COVERS SURFACE DENTS BUT NONE OF THE INTERIOR MATERIAL.

DR. INSURE

Most often dental insurance is only a *limited* benefit your employer provides. The rules depend on how much the employer (or the employee) pays into the policy. The higher the cost of the premium, the greater the dental benefits. The insurance company is in business to make a profit, and the company follows guidelines that determine how much money the policy is worth versus how much money will be paid out. This business concept is easy to grasp. What is not so easy to understand is how, when, and why your insurance provider could become your dentist.

Hmm...his plan covers teeth-not gums!

Here's How Dental Insurance Works

Insurance companies employ dentists as "hired guns" to review the dental diagnosis and treatment plans of their policyholders. In other words, Dr. Insure, hired by the insurance company and guided by the rules of the insurance plan, gives a medical summary of how any given patient should be treated. Based on this summary, the insurance company determines what parts of each dental procedure will and will not be paid. This system sets up a communication hurdle between patient and dentist.

No good health care provider wants to lose control of the overall care of a patient. And when the insurance company—from a distance—takes over a patient's diagnosis and care, the patient loses faith in the dentist. For example, imagine that a dentist gives a new patient a comprehensive dental exam and determines that she needs a crown. The patient has large decay under an old filling and needs the crown to protect and strengthen the tooth. She agrees and gets the crown. Her x-rays are sent to her insurance company along with the necessary paperwork.

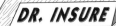

Dr. Insure examines her x-rays and paperwork and determines that the patient could have gotten by with only an amalgam filling. The insurance company makes a decision based on Dr. Insure's recommendations and delivers the final decree to the patient or dentist. The insurance company not only contributes a smaller percentage of the *cost* but also changes the *treatment*. It is only human nature to blame the person who delivers bad news. In this case, the bad news bearer is the dentist, so that's who the patient gets mad at and blames.

The patient assumes that either:

1. The dentist must be over-diagnosing to get more money from the insurance company.

    Or

2. The dentist didn't know what he was doing and made a mistake on the diagnosis.

What's Wrong with This Picture?

No matter what the patient assumes, she is bound to feel "ripped off." The insurance company has become the policy-holder's dentist. Dr. Insure reviews the patient's case in a remote corporate setting with no connection to the complex human being—the person whose name appears on the dental chart. The insurance company makes its decision and the dentist is caught in the middle. In reality, the dentist has no link with the insurance company or Dr. Insure or the patient's employer or the amount of benefits the patient's policy allows.

Sink Your Teeth into This: It has been our experience that the patient can usually get better results by calling the insurance company directly to discuss what dental procedures the policy covers and how much the company will pay. This is because you and your employer are the insurance company's clients; that is, you are the ones paying the insurance premiums. Sometimes complaints you have with your insurance may need to be channeled through your employer's Human Resource Department before being sent to the insurance company itself. Your dentist can give you the dental treatment information you need to have an informed discussion with your Human Resource Department and your insurance company.

Design a Dental Benefit Plan that Works for You

- ◆ Adopt a new attitude. Understand that your dental insurance is only a benefit.

- ◆ Read your insurance manual to familiarize yourself with the limits of your policy.

- ◆ Put your money where your mouth is. Understand that in order to receive the right care for healthy teeth and gums, you will need to make co-payments to supplement your dental benefits. Then you'll never be surprised or disappointed about your dental insurance coverage.

- ◆ Make sure that you have a happy dental home with a dentist you respect and trust and a dental team who treats you with respect and care.

- ◆ Decide whom you want to diagnose and treat your mouth—the insurance company or your trusted dentist? Ask yourself, "Who is working in my best interest? The insurance company's 'hired gun' dentist? Or the dentist I have personally selected?"

MOST FREQUENTLY ASKED QUESTIONS

These questions and answers may help clear up some of the confusion about dental insurance and money.

Q. *I have dental insurance and I don't understand why I still have out-of-pocket expenses for my dental work. Can you help?*

A. Your out-of-pocket expenses have everything to do with your company's dental plan and your zip code, not how much the dentistry costs. Your costs will depend on what type of dental insurance policy your employer selected for you. It is the old "you get what you pay for" principle. The more money your employer pays into premiums, the less out-of-pocket money you will have to pay.

Q. *My dentist won't send in my insurance claim so I have to do it. Is this a standard practice for most dentists?*

A. Not all dentists file insurance claims for their patients. The dentists who do, do it as a courtesy for their patients.

Q. *Why does teeth cleaning cost so much?*

A. A big part of the cost will depend on the state of your dental health and/or your state of disease. There are two types of cleanings:

- ◆ A PREVENTIVE CLEANING on a healthy set of teeth involves removing calculus, tartar, and debris from above the gum line, as well as checking for cancer, decays, and gum disease. The cleaning also includes polishing the teeth.

- ◆ A THERAPEUTIC CLEANING (or deep cleaning) costs more because the disease extends below the gum line. To do a deep (below the gum line) cleaning involves more time and skill and the proper equipment.

Q. *I haven't been to the dentist for a long time. The reason that I am dragging my feet is because I know it's going to be expensive. I really can't afford to go but my teeth are so bad. Do I dare make an appointment or is it too late?*

A. There must be a starting point. A good dental team will customize a step-by-step treatment plan to fit within your budget and extend over a period of time.

Believe it or not, you will feel so much better for getting the ball rolling. Once you get past this hurdle, you will see that it costs more money to neglect your teeth than it does to take care of them.

Q. *Why is it that there is never an end to working on my teeth? Is my dentist just trying to make money off me?*

A. You have to ask yourself a few questions in order to figure this out. Do you have lifestyle habits such as smoking, eating candy, sipping sodas, etc.? Decay and gum disease can be very active no matter how good a job the dentist does. If it is not a lifestyle problem, something else may be going on.

Here are some possibilities:

1. The dentist may be under-diagnosing your problems. This can happen when the dentist is afraid to tell you about all the dental work that you need.

2. The dentist didn't do a comprehensive dental exam from the get-go. So there was no long-term plan formulated for treating and taking care of your teeth and gums. As a result, you are getting the news piecemeal which explains why you are feeling as if *"there is never an end to working on my teeth."*

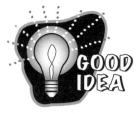

Direct dialogue between you and the dentist is a must! Ask for a comprehensive dental examination with a long-term, follow-up plan. Asking does not mean that you need to schedule all the treatment immediately, but it certainly prevents surprises.

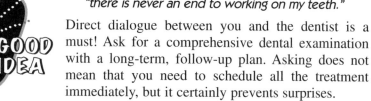

ALL-PAY, CO-PAY, WHO PAYS?

To clarify some of the confusion that surrounds dental insurance, here is a description of who pays what:

1. ALL-PAY: You pay the entire cost of your dental appointment. The dental office processes the necessary papers, and the insurance company writes the benefit check directly to you. Some dental offices will process the insurance paperwork for you and others will have you do it.

2. CO-PAY: Your dentist receives a co-payment from you along with your dental benefits. How this works: When you get a dental procedure done that is not totally covered by your insurance company, you will pay the dental office the portion of the cost that your insurance does not cover for the procedure.

You need to know this information to avoid any surprises. Determine which option is available at your dental office—all-pay or co-pay? Remember, it is not always possible for the dental office to know *exactly* what your insurance company will be paying.

Q. *Why do dental fees vary so much? And why is my dentist more expensive than the dentist down the street?*

A. Dentists are prohibited by the Sherman Anti-Trust Law from discussing fees. This law was enacted to protect the consumer from the practice of setting prices. Dentists really don't know what the guy down the street is charging or why he's charging that amount. If you want to shop prices, make certain that you are comparing apples to apples or you won't get a fair comparison.

Q. *How does a dentist price his work?*

A. In some countries with socialized medicine, dental fees are the same from one dentist to another. In the USA, dental fees vary from dentist to dentist. As an example, Dr. Lee's dental fees are based on his time and ability, business and staff costs, and a determination of a reasonable profit. This determination includes:

◆ The level of his technical skills (which goes far beyond dental school training).

◆ The amount of time necessary to treat a patient's particular dental problem without cutting any corners.

◆ Use of a dental laboratory that produces superior work, using high-quality dental materials and supplies.

◆ Benefits for his patients include a pleasant dental experience, being treated exceptionally well, and receiving a high-quality product that will last for many years.

Q. *Why are so many people getting root canals today? Is this just a way for the dentist to make more money?*

A. There are several reasons why dentists are doing more root canals. More people want to save their teeth (rather than get them extracted). People are living longer which increases their chances of getting dental infections. And the root canal procedure has a long and predictable history. Additionally, thanks to advanced technology, the root canal technique has been refined.

Q. *My dentist referred me to a specialist. Will I pay more money if I go to the doctor I am being referred to? The reason I ask is because I wonder if my dentist gets a financial kickback for referring me.*

A. It is illegal for a dentist to get any kickback money for referring a patient.

Q. *Why won't my dentist let me make monthly payments to pay for my dental work?*

A. A dental practice is a small business with ongoing overhead costs. It cannot afford to carry patients on an installment plan. You will find this is true in most businesses. When you purchase an item or service you either pay cash, put it on your credit card, or get it financed through a financial institution. Ask your dentist if there is a dental financed credit card available.

Q. *My dentist told me that I need to see him every three months. Isn't that too often?*

A. It depends on your stage of infection. The three-month visit is based on scientific studies that prove it takes three months for bacteria to repopulate at a level of destruction that can cause bone loss. Your dentist and/or hygienist determines the frequency of your dental visits based on various information including

DEALS THAT ARE TOO GOOD TO BE TRUE

Here are a few dos and don'ts that may save you some money in the long run:

DO **BE SKEPTICAL** of one-hour deals that show before and after photos of a fantastic "Hollywood smile" makeover. Claims like this usually are not possible because each mouth is different. One size does *not* fit all.

DO **THE MATH.** Example: Braces advertised for $88 a month. Ask how many months the braces will be on the patient. And get it in writing. It could be that paying more from the start (using the services of a highly recommended dental professional) actually turns out to be cheaper in the long run.

DO **READ THE FINE PRINT.** Example: Dentures advertised at a cost "too good to be true." When you read the fine print, you find out that the "too good to be true price" is for the "basic" denture and the "deluxe" denture and "the best" denture compute to about the same price as your own dentist will charge.

the state of your oral health and your lifestyle habits. In the long run, you will discover that maintenance and early detection are the least expensive routes.

Q. *Why won't my dental insurance pay for me to have my tooth replaced?*

A. It is likely that your employer purchased a dental plan that doesn't include replacing a tooth. And your policy may have a pre-existing condition clause. In other words, anything that happened before you started working with your present employer and enrolled in your current insurance company will not be covered. To be sure, read your insurance manual.

Q. *My dental insurance didn't pay as much for my crown as my dentist said it would pay. Why doesn't the dental office know exactly what my insurance covers and how much they are going to pay?*

A. There are thousands of different dental plans and each one has its own rules, guidelines, and regulations. It's your employer's and your responsibility to keep abreast of what's covered, what will be paid, and any changes that may arise. The dental office can only give you an *idea* of what the insurance company will pay.

Talk over your policy with your Human Resource Department. Insurance companies routinely change rules and prices as they see fit. There's no way a dental office could (or should) keep on top of those changes. That's where you, your employer, or your Human Resource Department needs to investigate and speak up.

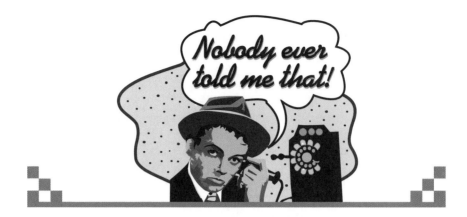

Nobody ever told me that!

- Your dental experience will be positive when you can: trust your dental professionals; know exactly what to expect; be confident that you can be in total control; and be confident that you will be numb or can be sedated in some way, if necessary.

- Have no fear. Today, modern pain control will help more than 90% of the people who could not get numb during a dental procedure in the past.

- If you compare the dental technology that exists today with a dental office of the 1930s, the progress is staggering. Available today are tools such as numbing gels, anti-anxiety medication, local anesthetics, nitrous oxide, oral sedation, and intravenous sedation, to name just a few. In the 1930s, there was only novocaine (and, for some people, whiskey).

- Pain is real and anxiety is real, but they are different issues. Anxiety must be dealt with on a person-by-person basis. Some people only need to know they are in control while in the dental chair. Others require distractions (such as watching TV or listening to music) or sedation such as nitrous oxide.

- There are four basic reasons why you can get a different diagnosis from one dentist to the next—time, training, experience, and integrity.

- When looking for Dr. Right, bring along your intuitive powers. You can judge a lot about a dental office from your first phone call. Was the person on the phone genuinely friendly and concerned?

- Make sure that Dr. Right gives you a comprehensive dental exam. We consider it a standard of care in dentistry.

- Here's an important question to ask the dentist when making a treatment decision: Is this the treatment you would recommend for your family members? Dr. Right will be happy to answer all your questions.

- During your professional teeth-cleaning appointment, ask the hygienist if he or she is using a probing tool to check for gum disease.

- Not all dentists file insurance claims for their patients. The dentists who will, do it as a courtesy service.

SECTION II:

THE TOOTH KILLERS:
Hold Onto a Good Thing

I won't let go of a good thing !

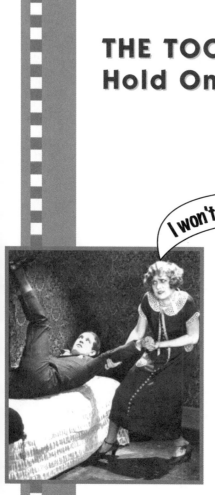

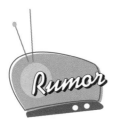

My gums and teeth must be healthy because I don't feel any pain.

Dental disease arrives as silently as a thief in the night. You may not feel pain until decay and gum disease have already reached an advanced stage.

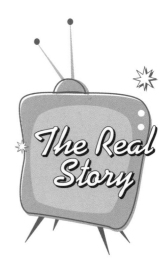

Three ways to lose your teeth

*E*verything we cherish takes some care and feeding. Your teeth need the same type of regular maintenance as your car, your garden, and your marriage. It is far healthier (and cheaper) to maintain your teeth and prevent the causes of tooth loss than it is to neglect your teeth and have to undergo costly, cumbersome, and painful repairs down the road. So treat your teeth like a cherished family heirloom and you should be able to hang onto them for a good, long time.

For most of us, the prospect of losing our teeth is terrifying. After all, tooth loss doesn't just affect our basic health and well-being. It also affects our good looks, the quality of our lives, and even our romantic prospects. Kissing, chewing, talking, and laughing—these are only a few of the vital functions that people who still have their natural teeth take for granted.

But the nightmare of tooth loss rarely occurs to us unless and until we start to feel mouth pain. If it don't *feel* broke, why fix it or even think about it?

Barring an accident like getting smacked in the kisser with a foreign object, there are only three ways to lose your teeth:

1. **Decay**

2. **Gum and bone disease**

3. **Problems with the way your teeth fit together**

The good news is that all three can be treated or prevented.

Section Highlights

- Anatomy of a tooth
- Breaking sweet lifestyle habits
- Detecting the silent tooth killer
- Living at high risk for gum disease
- Things that disturb bite harmony

SNEAKY DECAY:
Preventable Infection

*P*eople are often shocked to hear that tooth decay is an infection, and it is transmissible. Yes, you can catch it *from* someone and you can pass it *to* someone else.

Cavities occur for a variety of reasons, but the tooth killer in this scenario is a type of decay-causing bacteria. Of course we're taking some literary license to imply that "bad" bacteria has a goal—to reach the nerve and kill the tooth. Acid and bacteria penetrate the hard enamel covering of the tooth and, if left undetected, travel further into the tooth's soft dentin. As it journeys toward the nerve, the murderous bacteria multiplies, creating a destructive, decaying path. Fortunately, this toxic journey takes time. Decay doesn't destroy a tooth overnight.

Prevention, Intervention, or a Last-ditch Effort

Prevention: If the tooth is kept clean and free of plaque and bacteria is removed daily, tooth decay never has a chance to get started.

Intervention: If bacteria sneaks in and penetrates a path through the tooth's enamel, decay can still be stopped before it ever has a chance to do serious damage. The cavity can be replaced by a dental material that seals the tooth and helps prevent future problems.

Last-ditch effort: If the bacteria is left untreated and allowed to penetrate the tooth all the way down to the nerve, a root canal and crown are the only ways to save the tooth.

Decay is global: Decay has no ethnic or gender preferences. The common cold is the only infection more "common" than decay. But thanks to advances in

SIX INEXCUSABLE EXCUSES FOR AVOIDING THE DENTIST

1. I can't take time off from work.
2. I'm feeling no pain.
3. My teeth are so bad, I'm embarrassed to go to the dentist.
4. I'm afraid I will need a lot of dental work.
5. It costs too much money to go to the dentist.
6. I'm going to make an appointment tomorrow (and tomorrow never comes).

TEETH 101: WHAT MAKES A TOOTH

*T*o paraphrase an old proverb, "you can't always tell a tooth by its cover." From the outside, the tooth doesn't appear to be anything more than a hard, white substance. But when you look at the illustration below, you see that a tooth is really a complex network of nerves, tissue, fiber, and bone.

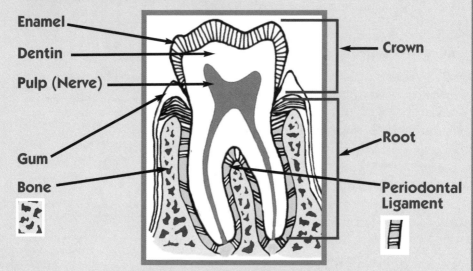

Enamel
Dentin
Pulp (Nerve)
Gum
Bone
Crown
Root
Periodontal Ligament

Enamel

The shiny, hard tooth covering. This is the strongest structure in your body.

Dentin

This structure essentially makes up the body of the tooth. It feels hard to the touch but it is actually porous and needs an enamel covering (or an artificial crown) to protect it from decay-causing bacteria.

Pulp

This soft tissue contains blood vessels, nerves and connective tissue. The pulp nourishes the tooth. If this tissue is damaged, your dentist or endodontist can remove it and save your tooth with root canal treatment.

Crown

This is the part of the tooth that is visible above the gum line.

Root

The root sits in the bone below the gum line.

Bone

The roots of your teeth are anchored by the bone in your jaw.

Periodontal Ligament

This tissue cushions both the tooth and the surrounding bone against the shock of chewing and biting.

Gum

Dentists call this the gingiva. It covers the bone surrounding your teeth and is important because it performs a big job—protecting against bacteria which causes gum/bone disease that can erode your jaw bone. Daily brushing and flossing keeps this soft tissue healthy.

dentistry and a greater emphasis on prevention, tooth decay has dramatically declined in the USA.

But make no mistake, the fight for improving dental health is far from over. Cavities still affect a major percentage of the population. Studies have found that 40 to 50 percent of U.S. children and adolescents in the 5-year-old to 17-year-old age group get cavities. For adults, more than 90 percent have evidence of past and present cavities.

Decay is sneaky. You generally won't feel any pain until decay has reached the nerve. When that happens, the infection has reached an advanced stage and is much harder to treat. Extensive and costly tooth repair will be necessary.

Where Does Decay Come From?

Decay occurs when your teeth are frequently exposed to foods and drinks that are high in starch, acid, and sugar—ingredients that feed or enhance the growth of decay-causing bacteria in your mouth. (Refined carbohydrates like crackers, white bread, and cereals act just like sugars and pose the same problem for your teeth.)

TOOTH DECAY MARCHES ON...

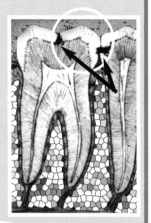

Moderate decay

In the illustration on the right, decay has penetrated the enamel and is entering the dentin.

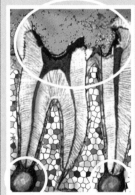

Advanced decay and abscess

In the illustration on the left, decay has destroyed the tooth and penetrated the nerve, which caused an abscess.

... IF LEFT UNTREATED

WHAT IS DECAY?

Despite modern advances in dental technology and science, a bit of mystery and controversy still surrounds the underlying causes of tooth decay. But here's what we do know:

Tooth decay begins as a bacterial infection. It is transmissible, but preventable. Decay-causing bacteria mixes with acid, food debris, and saliva to form a sticky substance called plaque. This plaque acts as a protective shield for bacteria, allowing it to grow and multiply. Over time, the acid produced by bacteria breaks down and eats a hole in the tooth's enamel. If left untreated, the acid and bacteria will eventually reach the soft dentin. When bacteria penetrates the dentin, infection can set in and spread to the tooth's nerve, unless the decay and bacteria are removed and the hole is sealed.

HOW FLUORIDE WORKS TO PREVENT DECAY:

1) Increases the strength of the calcium in the enamel to make it more acid-resistant.

2) Helps repair enamel that has been damaged by acids.

3) Kills decay-causing bacteria.

Because we all carry decay-causing bacteria in our mouths, everyone is at risk for cavities. Studies indicate, however, that if you have a history of tooth decay, you are probably at risk for more. That's because there are certain factors that increase your likelihood for tooth decay.

Your body's protective system may or may not be able to control the population of decay-causing bacteria (*Streptococcus mutans* and *Lactobacillus*). For example, if your protective system is effective, you can come in close contact with a person with a contagious disease and not get an infection. The goal for dental professionals and dental patients is to keep the number of bacteria below the disease-producing level in order to prevent decay.

The frequency and quality of your brushing and flossing can play a key role in preventing decay. Crooked teeth, braces, broken-down fillings, and improper dental work create overhangs, ledges, nooks, and crannies that catch food and make it tough to floss or brush teeth clean. This creates a breeding ground for bacteria and toxins. And don't be fooled into thinking that root canals or crowned teeth are invulnerable to decay—because they are not.

In dentistry, we *do* know that if you can control the population of the bacteria, you can stop decay. We *don't* know, however, 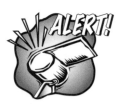 why one person's body is over-populated with bacteria, even with normal preventive measures, while someone else's body naturally keeps the bacteria population in check. The good news is that we have the ability to culture the saliva to confirm the quality and quantity of the destructive bacteria to determine who is at risk. To control

SALIVA: OUR NATURAL DEFENSE AGAINST TOOTH DECAY

Saliva is made up of water, proteins, electrolytes, mineral salts, calcium, and fluoride. A good flow of saliva is nature's way of washing food particles off the teeth and preventing decay. It is a natural buffer that stops acid from attacking the teeth. The calcium and fluoride in saliva help remineralize your teeth after an "acid attack." That's why people who suffer from dry mouth have such a tough time fighting decay. But saliva alone will not stop decay. Healthy lifestyle habits that help boost your immune system are equally important.

Streptococcus mutans and *Lactobacillus*, dental professionals can give you new therapeutic treatments and show you advanced cleaning techniques.

Other Factors that Increase Susceptibility to Decay

✔ **Your mother's health during pregnancy**
If your mom was sick and became feverish during the period your teeth were forming in-utero, your baby teeth may be less resistant to bacteria and decay.

✔ **Your health as a child**
High fever, disease, high intake of certain antibiotics, or too much or too little fluoride can cause soft teeth.

✔ **The anatomy of your teeth**
How the surface of your teeth is formed is very important. The depth and shape of the grooves in the biting surfaces of your molars will determine your chances of getting decay.

Signs and Symptoms of Decay

When it comes to decay, most signs and symptoms are so subtle only a trained dental professional can detect them. In many cases, decay cannot be detected by the naked eye. It takes technical help from an x-ray, digital image, intra-oral camera, or a special magnified eyewear (worn today by most technically up-to-date dentists) in order to ferret out decay. The benefits of early detection are many, including smaller restorations, lower dental costs, and the preservation of a larger number of your natural teeth.

Some Obvious Warning Signals of Decay

◆ Discoloration—Decay sometimes shows up as a brown stain

◆ Occasional sharp pain

◆ Throbbing pain that won't go away

◆ Sensitivity to sweets or to hot and cold foods and drinks

◆ A hole in the tooth

◆ A broken filling

◆ A cracked tooth

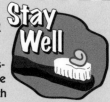

TRADE IN YOUR TOOTHBRUSH

Since decay is transmissible, *don't* share your toothbrush with anyone, especially your kids. Replace your toothbrush every one to two months and immediately after having a cold or the flu. This will prevent illness from lingering in your body.

Dental Prevention Pays Long-term Dividends

Let's get personal for a moment. How often do you brush and floss your teeth? Is it a chore you dread? Do you brush often but never floss? Or do you only floss when you get something caught between your teeth? When you were a tyke, did you perch in front of the TV and ignore Mom when she hollered, "Get in here and brush your teeth?" The truth is that we are all in the same boat. We all have teeth and we all have to take good care of them. But few of us really do. We're guessing that only at a dental convention will you witness the majority of people heading for the rest room after lunch to brush and floss their teeth.

On the bright side, it can be so easy and take so little time and effort to keep your teeth healthy—when they are already healthy. The key is to make brushing and flossing a habit—a part of your daily routine like combing your hair or washing your face.

Most people won't leave the house in the morning without a good tooth brushing, if only to avoid bad breath at work. The fact is that nighttime brushing is even more important. Our mouths naturally dry out while we sleep and our saliva is not around in abundance to fight off bacteria.

So here's where the nagging starts. You know that you're supposed to brush after every meal and floss at least once daily. But don't underestimate the importance of your brushing and flossing *technique*.

To make sure you're doing a good job of cleaning your teeth and gums, get some free advice from your dentist or hygienist during your regularly scheduled cleaning appointments. Like golf pros, they are trained to tell you what you're doing right and where your stroke could use a little more work.

Breaking Sweet Lifestyle Habits

It's surprising how many lifestyle factors and personal habits can increase your susceptibility to decay. Working with your dentist, you can control and, in many cases, conquer major risk factors that lead to "lifestyle cavities."

Ask yourself the following questions and find out how changing certain lifestyle habits can prevent tooth decay:

1. Do you continuously sip on carbonated sodas?

You're getting a "decay double whammy" if you drink sodas because of the high concentration of acid and sugar. This is why switching to sugar-free diet sodas doesn't really get you off the hook. And remember, drinking and sipping are two different actions. If you drink a soda and then rinse your mouth with water, there's a good chance your saliva will take care of potential decay problems. But if you sip sodas all day long, you are constantly feeding the bacteria in your mouth, allowing it to multiply and produce additional acid.

SODA SIPPING: ACID + SUGAR = A DECAY DOUBLE WHAMMY

Costly cosmetic dentistry was necessary to restore the decayed teeth.

 Our Recommendation: For you unrepentant sippers, try switching to sparkling water with a splash of sugar-free juice or a squeeze of lemon or lime. Or sip through a straw. This allows the beverage to bypass your teeth. If you must drink soda, use a straw and afterwards *immediately* rinse your mouth with water.

2. Do you chew sugared gum?

With every bite, chewing gum squirts sugar into and between your teeth. This "sugar rinse" causes bacteria to thrive in your mouth. Constant gum-chewing also has the effect of wearing your teeth down.

 Our Recommendation: Chew sugarless gum. Also ask yourself, are you chewing gum because it is a habit or because you are concerned about having bad breath? If bad breath is the culprit, you could have a serious condition that is causing bad breath. Discuss this problem with your dentist or hygienist.

3. Do you frequently suck on sugared mints or cough drops?

This is the biggest (and most ignored) decay culprit. People often overlook the fact that cough drops contain sugar (in fact, there is a teaspoon of sugar in each cough drop). Try to break the sucking habit by asking yourself why you do it in the first place. Is it for the purpose of refreshing your breath? Is it because you have a ticklish or sore throat? Or is it to help you with a dry mouth?

 Our Recommendation: If the cough drops are for your breath, stop trying to mask the bad odor and start looking for the cause. Ask your dentist and

■ ■ ■ ■ ■ ■ ■ ■ ■ ■ ■

HANDLE WITH CARE!

YOUR TEETH ARE NOT BOTTLE OPENERS

Teeth are at risk also from damaging habits that can cause chips and cracks.

Do not:

✔ Bite open potato chip bags.

✔ Use your front teeth to open bobby pins or barrettes.

✔ Bite your fingernails.

✔ Open nail polish (or any bottle for that matter) with your teeth.

✔ Chew on ice cubes, popcorn kernels, or pens and pencils.

✔ Use your teeth to bite thread or fishing lines.

■ ■ ■ ■ ■ ■ ■ ■ ■ ■ ■

hygienist if the odor is coming from your teeth or gums. If cough drops soothe your throat, make sure you visit your physician. You may have sinus drainage or allergies.

4. Do you frequently eat hard or sticky candy?

Candy that's hard or sticky tends to get lodged in the grooves and spaces between your teeth. Unless you brush and floss it out immediately after eating, the candy sticks to your teeth and becomes a sugar feeder for the bacteria in your mouth.

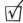 **Our Recommendation:** For candy lovers, chocolate is a better choice. It doesn't stick to teeth and can be washed off easily with water.

5. Do you chew tobacco?

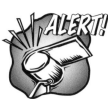 Several serious health problems can stem from chewing tobacco. One is oral cancer. Another is tooth decay. Because the leaves are dipped in molasses, chewing tobacco contains a large amount of hidden sugar. The sugar feeds the decay-causing bacteria. Moreover, tobacco is grown in sandy soil and the final product ends up containing a fine pumice that grinds down teeth.

☑ **Our Recommendation:** Quit. That's a strong statement, we know, but it takes a strong effort to get the job done. Chewing (or dipping) tobacco contains higher levels of nicotine than cigarettes and is even more addictive. (Anyone who has quit smoking cigarettes may find that hard to believe, but it's true.) Various nicotine replacement products like patches, gums, and inhalers are now available and have proven quite successful for those committed to quitting.

If you absolutely can't quit, even though you understand the tremendous health risks, don't chew on just one side of your mouth. Nicotine works as a constant irritant on the tissues of your mouth. Those who chew frequently have "rippling" of the cheeks inside their mouth. This rippling looks similar to the skin of a plucked chicken. This can indicate either a pre-cancerous or cancerous lesion. When chewing, move the tobacco around, frequently repositioning it to different places inside the mouth.

6. Have you ever had a problem with bulimia or anorexia or acid reflux?

Although the connection between eating disorders and tooth decay is not widely known, we do know that stomach acid from frequent vomiting can be quite toxic to your teeth and can lead to severe erosion of the enamel. Belching and back-up of stomach acids associated with acid reflux can also erode tooth enamel. Once the acid hits the dentin, the destruction is rapid.

 Our Recommendation: A dentist can diagnose the condition and correct the deteriorating enamel, but he or she cannot treat the actual eating disorder (or acid reflux). Visit a physician and/or psychologist immediately to treat this serious medical problem.

7. Do you have "dry mouth"?

People suffering from "dry mouth" (the technical term is *xerostomia*) usually adopt lifestyle habits that are dangerous to their teeth. During the day, they often compensate for their lack of saliva by overusing sugary mints, cough drops, and gum. At night, dry mouth often disturbs sleep by creating a tickle in the throat that causes coughing. When this happens, people often will pop cough drops or mints into their mouths and then fall back to sleep. The sugar sits and feeds bacteria for the rest of the night, which, in turn, can cause swift and rampant decay.

 Our Recommendation: Sip water constantly. Ask your pharmacist for over-the-counter mouth sprays. Talk to your dentist about prescribing fluoride tablets, and use them in place of sucking on cough drops or mints. You may also want to consult your physician to see if any medication you are taking is causing this condition.

PREVENTION IN THE 21ST CENTURY

Saving teeth has always been the first mission of dentistry. As we enter the 21st century, new dental technologies with cavity-sensitive detection devices will play a larger role in prevention. Dentists will place an increased emphasis on early detection and identification of high-risk patients.

THE FUTURE

GOOD IDEA

Dentists will also have the ability to accurately monitor and control the levels of Streptococcus mutans (the decay-causing bacteria) with a simple saliva test. If you experience frequent decay, ask your dentist if you need a *Strep mutans* saliva test.

Also on the horizon are new remineralization treatment therapies which are being developed for application in the dental office or prescribed for at-home use. There will also be advances in commercial toothpastes, mouth rinses, and therapeutic chewing gums that will help control decay. The 21st century certainly promises bigger, healthier smiles.

GUM AND BONE DISEASE:
The Silent Tooth Killer

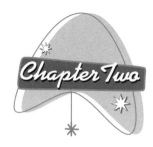

Chapter Two

*O*ne of the most pressing health issues we face today is gum and bone disease. For adults it is the major cause of tooth loss.

In 1998, an explosion of new medical research linked gum disease to other diseases in our body. It was revealed that gum infections may contribute to the development of strokes and heart disease; increase the risk of premature, underweight babies; and pose a serious threat to people whose health is already compromised by diabetes and respiratory disease.

Gum and Bone Disease:
What Is It and What Causes It?

Gum disease is a transmissible, bacterial infection that can destroy the attachment fibers and supporting bone that hold your teeth in your mouth. Gum disease is a complex disorder involving the interaction between specific types of bacteria and the immune response of the person infected. If not treated in a timely fashion, gum disease can lead to total tooth loss. Both children and adults should be routinely checked for gum disease.

GINGIVITIS: DON'T IGNORE IT

Today, gingivitis is almost a household word. It often appears in newspaper ads or is heard in TV commercials. Generally the focus of the advertising is bad breath. However, the appearance of gingivitis in the mainstream media has reduced the significance of gingivitis as an early warning sign. Gingivitis can signal that it's time for a dental check-up. Gingivitis symptoms include irritated and sometimes mildly inflamed gums that may appear red and swollen or may bleed during brushing. And, yes, bad breath is another possible symptom.

Determining whether gum disease is present (or just on the way) requires an evaluation by your dentist or hygienist. Red, puffy, irritated gums may also be due to a variety of problems—stress, medication, infrequent mouth care, or too few professional cleanings. Gingivitis can be reversed with professional cleanings and good daily mouth care. Why play guessing games? If the symptoms are present, don't take any chances. Let a dental professional diagnose and treat the real problem.

The bacterial plaque that causes gum infection is a sticky, colorless film that coats the teeth. Some types of bacteria are more difficult to fight than others. The stubborn variety pushes itself below the gum line and creates "pockets" between the gums and teeth. These pockets harbor trapped bacteria and plaque. If the plaque is not properly cleaned off, bacteria-laden tartar forms and hardens on the teeth, and the bacteria release toxins that irritate the gums. If the disease progresses, the pockets move deeper into the bone until no supporting gum tissue or bone is left. This process can systematically destroy the gums and bone. This loss of bone and teeth causes the face to sink inward and look many years older than its real age.

Immune System Factors Contribute to Gum Disease

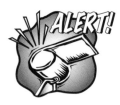

Dental disease, unlike other systemic diseases or certain heart diseases, cannot be reversed with only lifestyle changes. We cannot heal ourselves of decay or bone loss without the help of a good dental team. The infection must first be mechanically removed before you can depend on lifestyle changes or a strengthened immune system to keep decay or gum disease in check.

A certain percentage of people—about 15 to 20 percent—have immune systems that overreact to the bad bacteria in their mouths. When this overreaction occurs, the immune system attacks and breaks down the connective tissue that surrounds the tooth which leaves a path for the bacteria to travel into the bone and root of the tooth (see the illustration below). If you've ever played Pac-Man®, you understand how this works. The immune system chases the bacteria to kill it and, in so doing, also destroys bone and tissue. This destruction is not predictable and can occur sporadically. Please keep in mind that the body's immune system is extremely complex. We are deliberately oversimplifying the dental process of gum and bone disease for the sake of clarity.

None of us know if we are part of the 15 to 20 percent because we can't usually feel or notice the onset of gum and bone disease. But a qualified dentist who gives you a comprehensive exam can monitor any changes in your mouth and teeth. The dentist can then give you individualized treatment specific to the condition of your mouth.

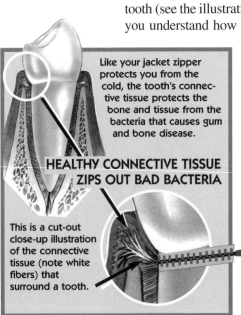

Like your jacket zipper protects you from the cold, the tooth's connective tissue protects the bone and tissue from the bacteria that causes gum and bone disease.

HEALTHY CONNECTIVE TISSUE ZIPS OUT BAD BACTERIA

This is a cut-out close-up illustration of the connective tissue (note white fibers) that surround a tooth.

Life circumstances and lifestyle choices can determine whether you will ever get gum disease. The presence of other illnesses or diseases can also affect your gums. For instance, diabetics need to take special care of their teeth and gums because they are more prone to infections of any kind. Genetic predisposition can also play a critical role in gum infections.

Are You Living at High Risk for Gum Disease?

Let's look at some lifestyle and life circumstance risk factors:

- ◆ SMOKING—Numerous studies show that smokers have more gum disease. Smokers and chewing tobacco users have higher levels of tartar in the mouth and experience more tissue irritation, which makes their gums more susceptible to disease. Not only do tobacco users have more bone loss, but they also heal less quickly than non-smokers.

- ◆ STRESS—Going through some tough times? We know there's a link between stress and dental health. When our immune system is stressed, it's difficult to fight off the bacteria that cause gum infections.

- ◆ DENTAL NEGLECT—Prevention is the name of the game in fighting any kind of disease. Dental health is no different. Avoiding the dentist is a lifestyle choice and puts you at risk for the diseases associated with your mouth, teeth, and gums.

- ◆ HORMONES—Hormonal changes in pregnant women and women taking birth control pills affect the gums and cause sensitivity that may make them more susceptible to gum infection. Many women report a higher incidence of bleeding gums during pregnancy.

WHAT HAPPENED TO AUDREY'S SMILE
FROM HIGH SCHOOL TO AGE 42?

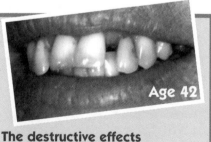

Age 42

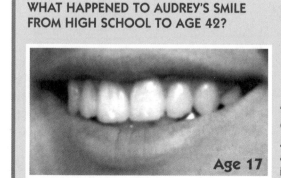

Age 17

**The destructive effects
of gum and bone disease.**
Audrey's lifestyle choices—smoking
and dental neglect—were key factors
in altering her beautiful smile.

TWO STAGES OF BONE LOSS

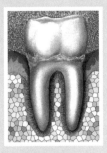

At this early stage, if the progression of bone loss is stopped and there is still enough bone to hold the tooth, the tooth can be saved.

BONE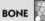

ADVANCED BONE LOSS

When there is not enough bone to hold the tooth in place, the tooth must be extracted.

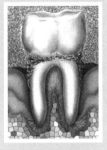

◆ **MEDICATIONS**—Certain drugs may affect the gums and cause swelling or dry the flow of saliva in the mouth. Dry mouth increases plaque build-up and leads to difficulties in brushing and flossing, which creates a greater risk for gum disease.

◆ **CLENCHING OR GRINDING YOUR TEETH**—These habits put abnormal stress on the teeth and can also put stress on the supporting structures of the teeth—the gums and bone.

◆ **POOR DIET**—Diet, to some degree, can make your gum tissue vulnerable to infection and resistant to proper healing. Gums need nutrients too! What you eat and the vitamins you take have an effect on your gums.

So what's the bottom line? If you are already practicing a healthy lifestyle and involving your dental team, chances are you are taking good care of your teeth and gums. Bravo!

The Signs and Symptoms of Gum Disease

Gum disease is often chronic and rarely gives any advanced warning that destruction is taking place. That's why it is necessary to get dental check-ups at least every six months. Keep in mind that healthy gums don't bleed. When they do, it signals, at the very least, a minor, reversible problem.

WHAT YOU DON'T SEE CAN HURT YOU!

Arrow indicates where bone *should* begin.

Patient's bone line.

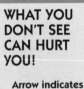

This digital image shows the patient's bone loss. Always ask to see your x-rays.

As you have probably learned by now, most dental diseases progress silently and gum disease is no exception. Some people will experience no warning signs or discomfort until the gum infection has progressed directly to the bone. With advanced bone loss, there isn't a prayer that your natural tooth can be saved. The good news is that new information about how gum disease works has led to a variety of new treatment options that increase the chances of controlling or even arresting the disease.

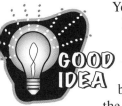

Your gums may be bleeding and you just haven't noticed it. Next time you floss your teeth, do a self-examination. Gently slide your floss below the gum line and check for blood on the floss. You can easily get below the gum line if you hug the tooth with the floss.

Keeping Your Gums in Shape

You are the key player on the hygiene team. If you don't do daily brushing and flossing, the rest of your dental team (the dentist and the hygienist) is playing shorthanded. And sometimes even with everyone fighting the good fight, stubborn bacteria and plaque will require some new maintenance techniques for battling gum infection. Section VI has in-depth cleaning tips and techniques that will help you beef up your daily mouth care routine.

When gum disease is present, your dentist or hygienist may give you a personalized mouth care routine and recommend that you:

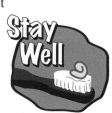

1. Reduce the length of time between dental appointments. Switch your regular six-month dental check-ups and cleanings to every three to four months.

DO A VISUAL EXAM AND A PERSONAL ASSESSMENT

Pull your lips up (and down) to reveal your gums and check your mouth:

- Do your gums look red and swollen or feel tender?
- Is a "pink color" noticeable on your toothbrush?
- Are your gums bleeding?
- Do you think that your teeth are protruding or does it seem that they are flaring out when they weren't before?
- Is pus or blood present between your teeth?
- Do you have persistent bad breath?

- Do your teeth hurt while chewing?
- Have you noticed an unpleasant taste in your mouth?
- Is there an "itchy feeling" in your gums?
- Do you feel any sensitivity to hot and/or cold foods or liquids?
- Push your teeth back and forth. Do they feel wobbly or loose?
- Can you see increased space between the front teeth?
- Do you feel more tired than usual or are you experiencing a loss of energy?

■ ■ ■ ■ ■ ■ ■ ■ ■ ■ ■ ■

ASK A PROBING QUESTION

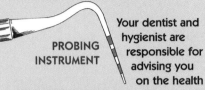

PROBING INSTRUMENT

Your dentist and hygienist are responsible for advising you on the health and condition of your gums. If your dental care provider is not using a dental probe during your routine cleanings and there is no mention of the health of your gums, it is time to consider a new dental home. How will you know if they are probing and measuring for pockets of gum disease? Be sure to ask.

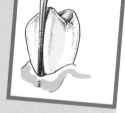

The illustration above shows use of probe to detect gum disease.

■ ■ ■ ■ ■ ■ ■ ■ ■ ■ ■ ■

2. Get in the habit of carrying floss and a toothbrush in your purse or backpack.

3. Brush and floss after eating lunch. You can do this at work or school. There's no law that says flossing can only be done at home.

4. Switch to an electric toothbrush, water irrigation system, or other specialized mouth care tools that will increase brushing quality and efficiency.

5. Use an antibacterial mouth rinse.

The Prevention, Diagnosis and Treatment of Gum Disease

The dentist is the first line of defense in treating your gum condition. The gums are primarily responsible for your overall dental health.

If gum disease is diagnosed, the dentist will initiate a treatment plan. This plan will start with aggressive, below-the-gum line cleanings and will include an individualized maintenance regime. For advanced gum disease, thorough dental cleanings and scalings and improved mouth care techniques are not always enough to keep the infection in check.

If surgery or special procedures are necessary, your dentist may feel more comfortable referring you to a *periodontist*—a dentist with advanced training who specializes in treating gum disease.

Gum disease is not curable, but it is treatable and, in most cases, controllable.

◆ If you are diagnosed with pockets in the gum tissue around your teeth that are greater than three millimeters, the recommended treatment is usually a non-surgical perio-therapy program. The severity of the infection will determine the length of the therapy. The treatment may require several visits.

The goals of the treatment are to:

1. Stop the bleeding.
2. Eliminate bacteria.
3. Shrink the gum pockets.

The dentist may prescribe antibiotics or insert antibiotics (*tetracycline*) and anti-microbials (*chlorhexidine, Ora5®*) directly into the gum pockets.

◆ If, after treatment, the pockets around the teeth do not shrink significantly or are too deep—five millimeters or more—surgery is sometimes necessary to remove the tartar, reduce the pocket, and arrange the tissue into a shape that will be easier for you to keep clean.

Following gum therapy, your gums and your mouth care should be carefully monitored at three-month to four-month intervals along with frequent, professional cleanings. When it comes to gum disease treatment success, maintenance and a conscientious mouth care routine are the keys to lasting health.

New 21st Century Gum Therapies

What's on the "perio-horizon?" During early stages of gum disease, special mouth rinses and toothpastes with anti-microbials are often used to control or destroy microorganisms. With gum disease as a major oral health problem, even more breakthrough products are on the way.

It also appears that the immune system plays a gigantic role in the fight against gum and bone disease.

ALL IN THE FAMILY

Are you saying that you can catch gum disease from another person? That's what people ask in disbelief when we tell them that gum disease, like decay, is transmissible. Research shows that the bacteria in gum disease can be transmitted through saliva. More often than not, it gets spread from one family member to the next—either parents to children or between couples.

That's why if one member of the family has gum disease, we recommend that the entire family see a dental professional for a gum screening. Some people are more susceptible to gum disease than others. It's likely that a genetic predisposition exits. If your parents have lost their teeth due to gum disease, are you destined to follow suit? Take it as a warning. Although your risk may be higher, it may not be inevitable.

WHAT ABOUT THOSE POOCH SMOOCHES?

Yup! We are suggesting that you may be at risk for catching gum disease from your dog or cat. The build-up of plaque and tartar in a pet's mouth can cause gum disease. Man's best friend needs a daily tooth-brushing routine too. If you own animals you probably already know this. Veterinarians have been able to educate pet owners about the link between Fido's gum disease and heart disease and other systemic diseases better than most dentists have done for their human patients. In fact, we know people who take better care of their pets teeth than they do their own teeth.

When researchers establish who is at risk and how and why the destruction occurs, then new treatment procedures and proven systems can be created and tailored to individual needs.

Ask your dentist (or periodontist) for more information on what's new, what's currently available, and what's appropriate for you. But remember that, right now, there's nothing so powerful that it will replace your mouth care cleaning routine. Oral hygiene is a lot like housekeeping—even with all our modern cleaning gadgets and high powered vacuums, we still have to sweep in the corners.

BITE BONUS:
If the Tooth Fits,
It Can Wear for a Lifetime

*T*he third way to lose your teeth is to have teeth that do not fit together properly. Our facial muscles, our teeth, and our jaw joints were created to work in harmony and balance for proper chewing and swallowing. A bite that is out of sync puts a strain on the teeth, the *temporomandibular joints* (TMJ), and facial muscles. When this happens, some people begin to clench and grind their teeth which causes a cycle of damage to teeth, jaw joints, and gums. The dental term for clenching and grinding is *bruxism* and people who clench are called "bruxers."

Why Bite Harmony Is So Important

Have you ever stopped to contemplate why only the lower jaw moves? This is because the upper jaw is part of the skull and is stationary. In fact, the lower jaw moves in many directions—up and down, side to side, front to back, etc.

When your bite is not in harmony, the poor fit can cause lower jaw movements which can totally destroy your natural teeth (as well as crowns and bridges) and can worsen the problem of teeth not fitting together properly.

Don't underestimate the power of your bite. Studies show that the strongest recorded bite strength was 975 pounds-per-square-inch (PSI) over a period of two seconds. The average chewing force may range from 55 to 286 PSI. This is an incredible amount of pressure isolated in one small area.

If an uneven bite is not properly addressed, teeth are at risk of breaking or wearing down to the gum line. To compensate for an uneven bite, clenching and grinding become continuous habits. Generally, people are not aware that they

TOOTH DAMAGE:

Tooth damage happens slowly over a long period of time and becomes noticeable only after teeth have become:

✔ Cracked   ✔ Worn
✔ Broken   ✔ Loosened
✔ Sensitive   ✔ Spaces between

WHY IT'S IMPORTANT THAT TEETH FIT TOGETHER PROPERLY

MISSING TEETH CAUSE PROBLEMS

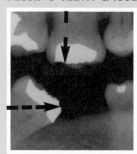

This digital image shows how the upper tooth is dropping to fill the space below.

The lower back tooth is collapsing into the empty space. The tooth may continue to fall forward until it is no longer functional.

A BITE OUT OF HARMONY CAN CAUSE CLENCHING AND GRINDING

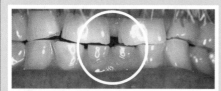

George's clenching and grinding has caused extreme wear on his teeth. Notice that the lower front teeth are almost worn down to the gum line.

have this destructive misalignment until they visit the dentist. A routine dental exam will reveal telltale wear and tear on the teeth.

Things that May Disturb Your Bite Harmony:

- ◆ Injury to the jaw
- ◆ Shifting teeth due to gum disease
- ◆ Crooked or misaligned teeth
- ◆ Arthritis in the jaw or jaw joint
- ◆ Ill-fitting dental work
- ◆ Missing teeth

Treatment for a Bite Out of Harmony

There is no cut-and-dried treatment plan for a bite that's out of harmony. Not every dentist is experienced in treating TM joint dysfunction problems. Ask how many cases your dentist has treated. And not everyone needs to be treated for a bite disorder. There are many variables and factors that come into play. Your individual situation should be carefully examined and discussed with your dentist before any treatment is started.

WHEN TEETH DON'T FIT TOGETHER PROPERLY

A variety of treatments may be recommended and may include:

- ✔ **A dental appliance (night guard)**
- ✔ **Posture training**
- ✔ **Ultrasound and jaw exercises**
- ✔ **Orthodontics**
- ✔ **Restorative work to correct more serious bite problems**

In some cases, the jaw joint becomes so severely damaged that surgery is required. Most professionals agree that surgery or any invasive procedure on the TM joint should be considered an absolute last resort.

Consider this:

- ✔ What is the status of your overall health?
- ✔ Are you under a lot of stress at work or at home?
- ✔ How serious is the damage to your teeth?
- ✔ Is there a predictable treatment outcome?
- ✔ Does the treatment justify time and cost?

Some people can live a lifetime with a bite disharmony, feel no pain, and show no wear on their teeth, while others simply cannot tolerate any bite discrepancy.

Sink Your Teeth into This: The verdict is still out on the perfect treatment plan. However, we *do* know that if teeth are worn, broken, or in any way damaged and no longer function correctly, they need to be restored to proper function.

If an incorrect bite involves facial pain or headache, we recommend starting with a conservative, non-invasive treatment. The dentist may advise you to wear a dental appliance similar to a retainer at night.

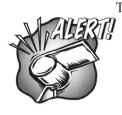

This is considered a conservative treatment because although the appliance is meant to alter your bite, it poses no physical risk. If it doesn't work, you throw the appliance away. Surgery, on the other hand, is not easily undone and should only be contemplated as a last resort.

We are not, however, suggesting that you procrastinate on treatment. Just take your treatment one step at a time.

Prevention Measures and Lifestyle Changes

Clenching and grinding can wear down and destroy your teeth. Self-care treatment is a necessary and important step that will enhance the effectiveness of other types of treatment.

Here are some measures your dentist will likely recommend:

- ◆ Keep your teeth apart. Teeth should come together only when eating or swallowing.

OUCH! ABOUT FACIAL PAIN

Up to 80% of facial pain from clenching and grinding teeth is caused by your facial muscles and not by the joints in your jaw. The facial muscles get overworked and react by going into muscle spasms (similar to a "charlie horse") which can cause an incredible amount of pain. These muscle spasms range from mild to severe and are often disguised as headaches. Only a small percentage of people who suffer with facial pain discover that the problem is caused by the TM joint.

Most people don't realize that teeth were not meant to be touching at all times. Give yourself a new mantra to chant: "lips together, teeth apart."

◆ When you catch yourself clenching your teeth, open your mouth slightly and rest the tip of your tongue between your teeth.

GOOD IDEA

◆ Stand tall. When you practice good posture, you will be practicing good jaw posture.

◆ Eat soft foods as a temporary measure to help rest your jaw.

◆ Manage stress. Stress will take a toll on your mouth. Daily stress management is a good idea for everyone, but it is especially helpful for people who clench and grind their teeth.

◆ Hot baths, massages, aerobic exercise, meditation, and yoga can all relieve stress and help restore harmony to your jaw joint and muscles.

◆ Don't chew gum or eat crunchy or chewy foods that can overwork the TM joints.

TMD: WHOM DO YOU CONSULT?

People who have TMD (*Temporomandibular Disorder*) often mistake their headaches for migraines and go to their physicians for help. Most medical doctors, however, are not trained to diagnose teeth and mouth-related pain. In some cases, a physician may decide that a CT Scan or MRI is necessary to rule out a tumor. Before undergoing costly medical tests and procedures, ask your physician whether it would be prudent to visit your dentist to make sure the pain is not being caused by TMD.

Signs and Symptoms of TMD

◆ A pattern of frequent headaches that occur at the same time each day

◆ Sore, stiff muscles around your jaw when you wake up

◆ Clicking and popping noises in your jaw

◆ Difficulty chewing food

◆ Difficulty opening your mouth while eating or yawning

◆ Sensitive, broken, worn, loose or missing teeth

◆ Earache without any sign of infection

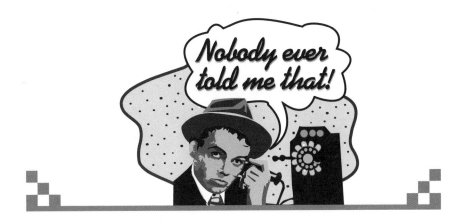

- A simple *Strep mutans* saliva test can determine whether you are at high risk for decay. Ask your dentist if you are a candidate.

- Never share toothbrushes. You can acquire the type of bacteria that causes decay and gum disease from another person or even from your pets.

- Diet sodas, cough drops, and chewing tobacco can cause tooth decay.

- Your diet, medication use, oral hygiene, and lifestyle habits will directly impact your problems with tooth decay.

- Throw away your old toothbrushes every one to two months, sooner if you've had a cold or the flu.

- When you lose teeth, you also lose the surrounding bone. The only purpose of this bone is to hold the teeth in your mouth. Without teeth, the bone disappears.

- Gum disease is treatable and, in most cases, controllable. Control the bacteria and you control the disease. Gum disease doesn't have to lead to tooth loss.

- Gum disease can lead to the spread of infection through your bloodstream, resulting in a loss of energy and fatigue.

- People mistakenly believe that their teeth must touch at all times. Not so. In fact, unless you are chewing, talking or swallowing, your jaw should be in a relaxed, slack position.

- Decay can occur at any age. You are never too old or too young to get decay.

- Imagine yourself in a plane flying over the Rocky Mountains. You are looking down on deep valleys and steep hills. The chewing surfaces on your back teeth, when magnified, look a bit like those mountains. These deep crevices will trap food and bacteria that can cause decay.

- Adults should ask their dentists if they need more fluoride. Fluoride treatments, gels, and tablets are available from the dentist.

There's a New Kid on the Block ...

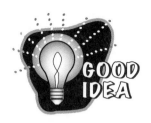

So far, we've been addressing the problems that result from an improper bite. You probably know people who have what looks to be a less-than-perfect bite and yet have no particular symptoms to complain about. Still others have ideal bites, but are almost always in pain. How's that possible?

- New research has shown that people with chronic headache pain **clench their jaws** about 14x more intensely than those without headaches.

- Migraine sufferers all have what is called "pericranial tenderness," meaning the musculature of their scalp is tender and sore, which is also a result of chronic nighttime jaw clenching.

This means that, regardless of their bite, some people may be chronic nighttime clenchers, resulting in headaches (some call it a regular "headachy" feel), neck pain, sensitive teeth, and even frequent migraine attacks.

Sometimes it's not just the bite that matters, it's the intensity of the **biting,** as well.

Your dentist has a new trick up his sleeve and it's called the NTI Tension Suppression System. The "NTI" is specifically designed to reduce the intensity of nocturnal clenching activity, regardless of the nature of one's bite. It's so effective that the FDA has recently approved it for the prevention of medically diagnosed migraine pain! You can learn more about the NTI at **www.HeadachePrevention.com**.

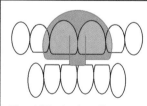

The NTI device fits comfortably on your two front teeth while you sleep.

SECTION III:

YOUR MOUTH:
The Gateway to Your Health

'Round the teeth, through the gums look out body here it comes!

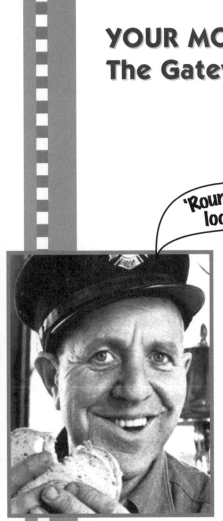

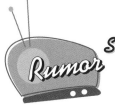

Rumor Staying healthy means eating right, frequent exercise, and regular medical check-ups.

Add regular dental check-ups to that list. Current research shows that dental check-ups are even more important than we thought. Gum disease has been linked to heart disease, low birth-weight babies, diabetes, and other systemic diseases.

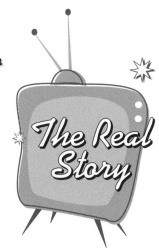

The Real Story

Get to the heart of the matter

"It seems clear that gum disease, far from being just an oral health problem, actually represents a significant health risk to millions of people."

Robert Genco, D.D. S., Ph.D.
Editor-in-chief,
Journal of Periodontology

According to the American Heart Association, cardiovascular disease is the leading cause of death for men and women of all ethnic groups.

Smoking, hypertension, obesity, diabetes, and high cholesterol levels are well-known risk factors for heart disease. However, new research is shedding more light on the strong link between gum and bone disease and cardiovascular disease.

A study published in the *New England Journal of Medicine* found that men with high levels of periodontal inflammation are at increased risk for heart attacks and may have nearly twice the risk for *fatal* heart attacks. Another study shows that the strain of bacteria found in gum disease can cause blood clotting when it enters the bloodstream. This blood clotting can contribute to the clogging of arteries.

Researchers believe that inflammation caused by mouth disease contributes to plaque build-up in the arteries. Moreover, there seems to be a connection between chronic inflammation of the gums and inflammation of the blood vessels throughout the body.

Section Highlights

Important new health information:

- ◆ Gum disease may travel to organs in your body
- ◆ How your medical condition influences dental treatments
- ◆ Infections and other mouth maladies

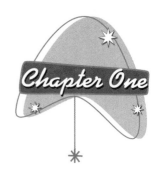

Chapter One

THE MOUTH-BODY CONNECTION:
New Health Information

*W*e tend to think that the dentist's only function is to help keep our teeth and gums healthy. What dentists have suspected for a long time is now confirmed—disease in the mouth is hazardous to your health. More and more medical research shows that a number of life-threatening illnesses may get their start from the bacteria associated with gum disease.

Most of us strive to live healthy lives—if we don't, we at least have the good sense to feel guilty about not trying hard enough. A large percentage of the population lives and breathes fitness. They aim high and get on target with power walks, a menu of body-pampering services, Feng Shui makeovers, and vitamin pumped smoothies. They eat only low fat foods, do regular breast checks, and lather on sunscreens. But what most fitness-driven consumers don't understand is the potentially deadly connection between diseases of the mouth, gum and bone, and overall health.

Medical research is saying that when we neglect our dental health, the devastating consequences directly affect how quickly we lose our health, our good looks, and damage our vital organs. And no yoga workout or biceps curls or cholesterol blasters can restore vitality when the body is compromised by gum disease.

The bottom line is that the mouth is the gateway to body and health. Your dentist acts as the gatekeeper, protecting you against gum and bone infection and preventing harmful bacteria from entering the bloodstream and attacking vital organs. That's quite a mouthful!

FLOSS OR DIE

The headline of a 1998 *USA Today* newspaper report—*Floss or Die*—explaining the link between gum disease and other diseases may not necessarily be an overstatement. In fact, two of the most common chronic diseases in the world—tooth decay and gum disease—are located within the walls of our mouth.

Left untreated, these oral infections can lead to the destruction of the enamel, root surfaces, dentin, ligaments, and jaw bones—not to mention tooth loss. Though quite serious, these conditions are not directly fatal. However, current studies show that complications from these oral diseases may destroy vital organs and may even lead to death.

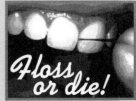

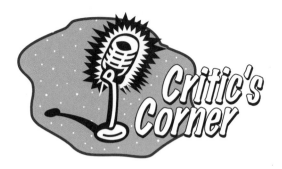

Pet Peeves

*T*he word is out from veterinarians to pet owners. But the pet owners never seem to get this information from their own physicians. Why don't medical doctors make the connection between oral health and total physical well-being? I'm looking at a Pfizer animal health brochure. The text reads: *"Dental care keeps more than your pet's teeth from going bad... Plaque builds up ... pockets form ... bacteria from the oral infection have a clear path to the animal's bloodstream and vital organs."*

Today, a large body of medical research suggests that gum disease, when allowed to run rampant, may spread throughout your body and threaten major organs. I don't know about you, but I have a few questions. Why don't medical doctors talk about this link between infection in the mouth and the rest of the body? People who seek help from their physicians for feeling tired and run-down aren't often diagnosed or referred to their dentists, even though their illness may be due to deep pockets of infection from their gums. Why not? Veterinarians are hip to the seriousness of gum infection and decay.

When someone wants to put off necessary dental work, he or she often says to the dentist, *"I'm not going to die if I lose my teeth. It's not like losing a kidney."* But now medical research reports that you *can* die from diseases associated with the bacteria in gum disease. Maybe that makes your toothbrush and floss your new best friends.

Next time you see your physician, ask him or her to take a dentist to lunch. Shouldn't the two professions (body doctors and mouth doctors) work together to serve our best interest?

BACTEREMIA

Bacteremia is a condition which exists when bacteria is introduced into your bloodstream. Once in your bloodstream, bacteria will travel to other parts of the body including your heart, joints, and lungs.

There are 300 species of bacteria that live in the mouth. Bacteria can be present for years before any disease or pain is ever associated with it.

Healthy Gums, Healthy Body

Diseases that link gum disease to bacteremia include:

- ✔ Heart disease
- ✔ Stroke
- ✔ Diabetes
- ✔ Respiratory disease

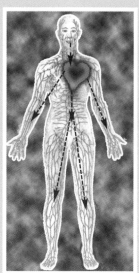

HAVE GUM DISEASE ... WILL TRAVEL.

Your dentist works to prevent infection in your mouth from entering the bloodstream and reaching vital organs.

Although bacteremia can occur during routine brushing or chewing, it usually is detected *after* dental procedures. This may sound alarming, but it's not meant to scare you from seeing the dentist. On the contrary, your dentist and hygienist are your best defense against bacteremia, because they can help you prevent a build-up of plaque and bacteria in your mouth.

A Dangerous Form of Bacteremia

Bacterial endocarditis is a severe life-threatening infection of the inner lining of the heart and valves caused by bacteremia. This bacteremia can come from other infected parts of your body. Though not common, it can also occur during minor dental procedures in which bleeding occurs.

DIABETIC ALERT: THE SWEET AND SOUR NEWS

New evidence shows that people with diabetes face a greater risk of gum disease than the general population. This is due to the fact that many diabetics experience fluctuating blood-sugar levels which causes a decrease in saliva production and, in turn, increases the risk of gum disease and decay. On the flip side, infections stemming from gum disease can actually increase blood sugar in the body, causing a host of diabetes-related health problems. Diabetics must keep their gums in peak condition, work extra hard on their brushing and flossing routines, and see their dentists regularly.

BEWARE:
SELF-INDUCED BACTEREMIA

It is true that dental procedures can cause bacteremia and the more infection you have, the more likely bacteremia will occur. However, many physicians and consumers don't realize that bacteremia can be self-induced. If you have gum disease with signs of pus and/or bleeding gums, bad breath or a foul taste in your mouth, bacteremia may occur while you brush your teeth, chew food, floss, or do any activity that applies pressure on the gums. The only way to avoid self-induced bacteremia or dental-induced bacteremia is to have healthy gum tissue.

Do You Have Risk Factors for Bacterial Endocarditis?

Before you undergo gum or bone treatment, be sure to notify your dentist if you:

✔ Had a heart attack recently.

✔ Are recovering from heart surgery.

✔ Take heart medication or anticoagulants.

✔ Have an irregular heart beat.

✔ Wear a pacemaker.

✔ Have had vascular surgery (replaced artery).

✔ Have an artificial heart valve.

✔ Have a history of rheumatic fever or heart murmur.

✔ Experience angina (chest pain).

✔ Had previous bacterial endocarditis.

Patients who are taking anti-coagulants, aspirin, garlic supplements, etc., should ask their dentist whether any special precautions should be taken prior to treatment.

If your dentist believes that you may be at risk for bacterial or infectious endocarditis, he or she may prescribe a precautionary round of antibiotics *before* performing any dental procedure.

Joint Replacement Surgery and Gum Disease

If you require joint replacement surgery, you must be in good health prior to surgery, and this includes infection-free gums. If not, you risk possible infection and a slower recovery resulting from bacteria adhering to the new joint replacement. In fact, many medical doctors will recommend that their patients complete any necessary dental work *before* joint replacement surgery. Once the joint replacement is finished, it is very important to stay on top of your oral hygiene to reduce the risk of gum-induced bacteremia. Your dentist and physician can provide you with more information.

Breathe Easier with Healthy Gums

The elderly, people who smoke, and those suffering from a weakened immune system are at increased risk for respiratory complications and diseases like bronchitis, pneumonia, emphysema, and chronic obstructive pulmonary disease.

And now it has been shown that gum disease—our old neme-sis—is also a significant risk factor for respiratory disease. In some cases, studies show that infections of the mouth are directly associated with respiratory infection. If you think you might be at risk for either gum or respiratory infection, it is time to get a complete gum evaluation.

Pregnancy, Gum Disease, and Your Baby's Health

Pregnant women with certain types of gum and bone disease have an increased risk of delivering low birth-weight babies. The more infected your gums and teeth become, the greater the chance that bacteria can travel through your blood stream to your fetus. The infection may cause an immune response that damages the tissue in the placenta and may even prompt premature labor, as well as a low birth-weight baby.

YOUR MEDICAL HISTORY AND YOUR DENTAL WORK

The practice of completing an in-depth medical history for the dentist is becoming more and more important especially as we age. And because health problems such as diabetes, arthritis, and heart disease all require medication, it is criti-cal for dentists to thoroughly screen their patients before prescribing any medication.

At your first appointment with a new dentist, carefully fill out your medical history chart. Information about your general physical condition, allergies, reactions to drug, the medications you are currently taking, medical conditions that require antibi-otic pre-medication, lifestyle habits that may affect your health, and previous dental work are all valuable pieces of information for your dentist.

HEADS UP! THERE'S GUM TISSUE ATTACHED TO THIS TOOTH!

Many Americans visit their dentist twice a year for a cleaning and general check-up. However, it is important to make sure that your dentist is also measuring and check-ing for gum disease and bone loss. No obvious bells or whistles will blow when gum infection begins and some dentists might not be looking for the early stages of gum disease. Early detection will dramatically lessen damage to the mouth and teeth and, as we are now learning, to the rest of your body. This is just another important rea-son why it is imperative that your annual dental exam focus, not just on your teeth, but also on your gums and bones.

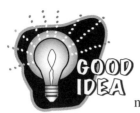

At every dental visit, update your medical chart and inform the dental team of new medical and dental information such as a change in medication, any upcoming surgery, a change in blood pressure, or new allergies.

No Secrets, Please

Good communication between you and your dental team begins with a complete health history. However, with any relationship, it's the little things that can mean a lot. Information you may think is meaningless can be vital for your dentist to know.

Here are a few examples:

◆ Do you have an allergy to latex? Dental professionals regularly wear latex gloves and use latex rubber dams.

◆ Do you have allergies to jewelry? Certain dental metals may need to be avoided.

◆ Do you have any oral or topical medication allergies (for example, iodine or penicillin)? If so, make sure the dental team knows.

◆ Do you easily gag? Let the dentist know because he or she may decide to alter certain procedures.

◆ Are you taking aspirin on a daily basis? If so, keep in mind that aspirin works as a blood thinner and you may bleed a lot more easily.

◆ Do you take birth control pills? This is important information when a dentist is prescribing an antibiotic because the medication may cancel out the birth control pills and stop them from working.

◆ Do you have anxiety attacks? If so, communicate this to the dental team. They can use a variety of techniques to relieve your anxiety.

◆ Have you ever had a reaction to a dental injection? If so, explain your reaction in detail to your dentist.

◆ Have you had cataract surgery? The dental team will give you protective glasses to wear during certain procedures.

◆ Do you have any physical limitations? Most dental procedures are done in a reclining position. Tell the dentist about feelings of claustrophobia, any back or neck problems, or any condition that won't allow you to recline. A pillow under your neck or back might be just what you need.

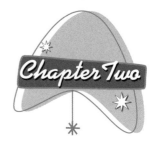

Chapter Two

ORAL REPORT:
Signs of Trouble

ORAL CANCER

Oral cancer accounts for about three percent of all cancers. As with many cancers, early detection can greatly increase chances of survival. Dentists are generally your first line of defense when it comes to detecting oral cancer. As part of your annual check-up, your dentist should perform an oral cancer screening beginning with your tongue—the most common site for oral cancer.

Unfortunately, oral cancer often goes overlooked until it has spread to the lymph glands and forms a knot on the neck. The risk is highest among people over 40 years of age who are heavy users of tobacco and alcohol. The average age at the time of diagnosis for oral cancer is about 60. Pipe and cigar smokers run a higher risk of cancer of the lip, and people who chew tobacco are at much greater risk for cancer of the cheek. Over-exposure to the sun also increases the risk of lip cancer.

ADVICE FOR ORAL CANCER PATIENTS
Radiation of the neck, throat, and jaw can cause serious dental complications. When possible, get a dental check-up (and any needed dental work completed) *BEFORE* radiation therapy because radiation will slow the healing process.

What the Studies Show:

- Smokeless tobacco may increase by four times the risk for oral cancer.
- A pack of cigarettes per day increases risk for oral cancer 4.5 times.
- Drinking up to six alcoholic drinks per day increases the risk 3.3 times, six to nine drinks per day increases cancer risk 15 times.
- Together the heavy use of tobacco and alcohol can make your risk of oral cancer up to 100 times higher than the rest of the population.

Four Signs of Possible Oral Cancer

1. A mouth sore that bleeds easily or fails to heal.
2. A lump, thickening, or soreness in the mouth, throat, or tongue.

3. Soreness or swelling inside the mouth that does not go away.

4. Difficulty in chewing, swallowing, or moving your tongue or jaw.

TYPICAL (and not so typical) ORAL AFFLICTIONS

Millions of people suffer with recurring, painful mouth sores. Canker sores are a common mouth malady, but generally do not represent a serious health problem. They can be effectively treated and sometimes even avoided. Canker sores are frequently confused with cold sores (fever blisters) but it's easy to tell the difference.

Canker sores (sometimes called "mouth ulcers") are not caused by a virus, so they are not contagious. The sores only occur inside the mouth. Bacteria in your mouth will often cause canker sores to become even more inflamed. Keep your teeth and gums clean.

Cold sores (also called "fever blisters") are caused by the herpes virus and are highly contagious. Cold sores frequently show up on the *outside* of the mouth on or near the lips. However, they can also appear inside the mouth.

Canker Sores

Canker sores usually start rearing their ugly heads when stress is at its highest. Some people are lucky and only get canker sores occasionally, while others (usually teenagers and young adults) suffer more frequent episodes.

Sometimes trauma from rigorous tooth brushing, biting your tongue or cheek, or hitting the inside of your mouth with a sharp or hard object can trigger a canker sore. Other possible causes include acidic foods, food allergies, the toothpaste ingredient SLS (*sodium lauryl sulfate*), stress, throat infections, digestive conditions, vitamin deficiencies, and even your parents since susceptibility to getting canker sores can be inherited.

Prevention

1. **Keep a food diary.** Nuts, peanut butter, seafood, wheat products, chocolate, and milk are foods that have been found to trigger canker sores.

2. **Read toothpaste labels.** Select a toothpaste *without* SLS. Try it for 30 days. It may make a difference. Also, be sure to brush gently.

3. **Decrease and manage your stress level.**
4. **Ask your dentist or hygienist for advice.** You may be biting or hurting the inside of your lip or mouth.

Treatment

☑ **Rinses and gels** that your dentist can prescribe. Or your pharmacist can recommend over-the-counter canker sore products.

☑ **ORA5®,** a product manufactured by Dr. Mac Lee, is an effective non-prescription medication available for the treatment of canker sores. Ask your dentist for more information or check Web page www.ora5.com.

Oral Thrush

Oral thrush (*candida albicans*) is an uncontrolled overgrowth of fungus (yeast) in the mouth. This is the same fungus associated with vaginal yeast infections. Thrush may be the result of an immune system compromised by illness, stress, or immune disorders such as AIDS or by circumstances in which the balance of normal microorganisms has been upset by the long-term use of antibiotics. Oral thrush is also associated with uncontrolled *diabetes mellitus* and with hormonal changes associated with pregnancy or the use of birth control pills.

Oral thrush is most common in infants, toddlers, and the elderly. Thrush is also higher for people wearing ill-fitting dentures and for those who suffer with "Dry Mouth Syndrome" (*xerostomia*).

Signs of Trouble

An examination of the mouth will reveal:

☒ White, creamy lesions in the mouth (usually on the tongue or inner cheeks).

☒ Tender, red patches underneath the lesions that may bleed.

☒ Pain and difficulty eating.

If you think you have oral thrush, call your physician immediately.

Treatment

◆ Good oral hygiene
◆ Warm salt water rinses
◆ Correcting ill-fitting dentures
◆ Prescription medication

■ ■ ■ ■ ■ ■ ■ ■ ■ ■

RADIATION THERAPY AND DRY MOUTH SYNDROME

Radiation therapy used to treat head and neck tumors damages the salivary glands as early as the first week of radiation which can cause Dry Mouth Syndrome. This opens the door to a host of other oral problems including oral infection and tooth decay. Often patients also experience great difficulty in speaking, eating, and swallowing.

■ ■ ■ ■ ■ ■ ■ ■ ■ ■

Discard your toothbrush once treatment has been completed and avoid using any over-the-counter mouth rinses or sprays that could upset the balance of microorganisms in your mouth.

Dry Mouth Syndrome (Xerostomia)

Most people don't realize that saliva provides us a vital service and comfort. Saliva is the main protective element for safeguarding against bacteria in your mouth. Salivary proteins protect your teeth by keeping them hard, they help repair wounds in the mouth, and they kill bacteria (and even some viruses).

Saliva also acts as a lubricant in your mouth. The lack of it (called Dry Mouth Syndrome) causes teeth to stick to the cheeks, making it difficult to speak and eat. When saliva runs short, it also becomes more difficult to keep your teeth clean because plaque and food stick to teeth which increases the chances for decay. In fact, this is the number one reason that people with Dry Mouth Syndrome get rampant decay.

Dry Mouth Syndrome can be the result of taking certain medications. More than 400 drugs, many of which are commonly used, can cause oral dryness. These include anti-cholinergic drugs, anoretics, antihistamines, anti-depressants, antipsychotics, antihypertensives, diuretics, anti-Parkinsonian drugs, and muscle relaxants. These drugs do not damage the structure of the salivary glands. They just inhibit the production of saliva.

Signs of Trouble

[X] Drinking large quantities of water without relieving the dry mouth

[X] An increase in decay

[X] An inability to wear dentures

[X] Difficulty chewing and swallowing food

[X] Loss of taste, especially bitter and sweet

[X] Mouth ulcers

Three Stages of Treatment

1. Dental consultation and preventive dental care
2. Dietary counseling
3. Moisture replacement including artificial saliva

Sjorgen's Syndrome

This chronic disorder primarily affects women between the ages of 35 and 55. It occurs when the body's immune system attacks the glands that produce tears and saliva. Individuals suffering with Sjorgen's Syndrome may also be afflicted with rheumatoid arthritis.

Signs of Trouble

The signs of trouble for Sjorgen's Syndrome include the same symptoms listed for Dry Mouth Syndrome. In addition, the following are three systemic symptoms of Sjorgen's Syndrome.

- ☒ Excessively dry eyes, nose and mouth
- ☒ Swollen glands
- ☒ Joint inflammation

Treatment

- ◆ Increase the production of saliva with an over-the-counter spray and/or chew sugarless gum.
- ◆ Moisten dry eyes with eye drops.
- ◆ Ask your dentist for treatment recommendations.

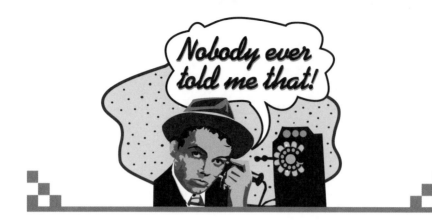

- Gum disease is a risk factor for heart and respiratory disease patients.
- If you are scheduled to have joint replacement surgery, you can help prevent a post-surgery infection by getting necessary dental work completed *before* surgery.
- When you suffer from gum disease, brushing or flossing your teeth, chewing food, or any activity that involves pressure on your teeth and gums puts you at risk for pushing harmful bacteria into your body.
- Infections that stem from gum disease can increase blood sugars in the body which can create serious health complications for diabetics.
- Pregnant women who have infected gums increase their risk for delivering premature or low birth-weight babies.
- The average age for diagnosis of oral cancer is approximately age 60.
- Dentists are your first line of defense for detecting oral cancer, which usually begins on the tongue.
- Smokeless tobacco may increase the risk of oral cancer by four times.
- Canker sores generally rear their ugly heads during the teen years. Stress is the main culprit.
- If you get canker sores frequently, try this 30-day test. Avoid using toothpaste with the ingredient SLS (*sodium lauryl sulfate*).
- If you are prescribed a long-term antibiotic, keep a watchful eye out for signs of oral thrush—a yeast infection inside the mouth. White, creamy patches inside the mouth may signal a problem.
- Dry Mouth Syndrome can be the result of a medication side effect. Consult your physician or dentist.
- Radiation therapy used to treat head and neck tumors damages the salivary glands. This damage can cause Dry Mouth Syndrome. When possible, get necessary dental work completed *before* radiation therapy.
- At every dental visit, update your dental team on any recent medications, surgery, or physical limitations.

SECTION IV:

YOUR CHILD'S DENTAL HEALTH:
From Womb to Wisdom Teeth

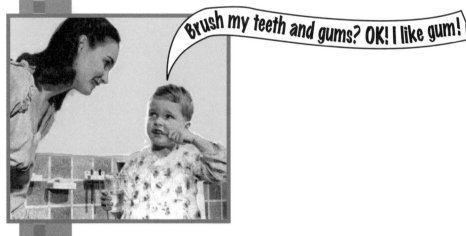

Brush my teeth and gums? OK! I like gum!

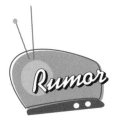

Rumor

But, Doc, they are only baby teeth. Why do we need to fix them?

The Real Story

Healthy baby teeth play an important role in your child's nutrition and in the development of self-esteem and social skills. They must serve the child until the permanent teeth come in at around age 10. That's longer than some people drive their cars!

Bringing up baby's teeth

*C*onsider this section the definitive "field guide" to your child's dental care—from womb to wisdom teeth. It is a fact that early prevention is key. But once your dental IQ is raised, you will also recognize that it is never too early (or too late) to lean on the wise guidance of a caring dentist and dental team. With that in mind, we organized the following information into age-specific sections, so you can jump in and get started, no matter how old your child is.

Childhood is a time of transition when children go from no teeth to baby teeth to adult teeth. And, at every turn, their behavior and personalities change. Nothing is predictable when it comes to children. Every mom and dad wishes they had a "how to" formula that would guide them through the numerous stages of their child's life. Fortunately, parents don't need to bring up baby's teeth alone.

Dental prevention in its purest form protects teeth that are immaculate, unspoiled, and without blemish or repair. Once teeth are "fixed," a cycle of dental repair and re-repair begins and continues for the life of the tooth. The best dentistry is no dentistry at all. In other words, prevention and early detection not only ensure a healthy dental future, they keep the child out of harm's way and give parents peace of mind, while saving time and money on costly dental procedures.

Section Highlights

What to do for your child's dental health:

◆ Before baby is born

◆ Birth to 2 years

◆ 3 to 6 years

◆ 7 to 12 years

◆ 13 to 18 years

◆ Calendar of dental visits

Chapter One

STARTING IN THE WOMB: Great Beginnings for Mom and Baby

*W*hen it comes to children's dental health, the best possible time to start the care and feeding of your baby's mouth is while you are pregnant. At around three weeks, before you are even sure you are expecting, your baby's mouth begins to form. During week five or six, the "buds" that develop the primary (baby) teeth appear.

At birth, your baby has a full set of primary teeth under the gums, as well as a set of permanent teeth in varying stages of development. And when the baby teeth start to emerge, between six and 12 months, it is time to visit the dentist. Prevention that begins at the very beginning increases the odds that your baby's teeth will be healthy for a lifetime.

Precautions for Expectant Moms

A woman's gum tissue changes during pregnancy. First-time mothers tell us, "I knew my body was going through major changes, but I didn't realize my mouth was too!" During pregnancy, a surge of hormones (mainly estrogen), creates an increase in the plaque build-up on the teeth. The tissue in the lining of the uterus is almost identical to the tissue in the mouth. When one changes, so does the other. If the pregnancy plaque isn't removed, it may cause a gum condition called "pregnancy gingivitis."

Infected Gums Can Affect the Fetus

The more infected your gums and teeth become, the greater the chances are that bacteria will travel through your bloodstream to your fetus. This causes an immune response that damages the tissues in the placenta and sometimes prompts premature labor and/or a lower birth-weight baby.

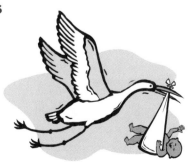

■ ■ ■ ■ ■ ■ ■ ■ ■ ■

PREMATURELY BORN BABIES

A premature baby's teeth may not have had a chance to get the full benefits of pre-natal development. This can lead to dental complications. *Enamel hypoplasia* is the main concern. This condition causes teeth to be softer, less smooth, more prone to chipping, and prone to turning brown. So, it is especially important for premature babies to see a dentist as soon as the first tooth appears.

■ ■ ■ ■ ■ ■ ■ ■ ■ ■

Do a little investigating. Pull your lip down and inspect your mouth and gums for:

- ✔ Puffy and red gums
- ✔ Tender and bleeding gums while brushing and flossing
- ✔ White, sticky plaque around the teeth and gums

The Best Ways to Care for Your Teeth

Your daily brushing routine is very important during your pregnancy, but some moms complain that brushing their teeth in the morning makes their "morning sickness" worse. If that is the case for you, rinse your mouth with water or anti-plaque and fluoride mouthwash. Later in the morning, after the "morning sickness" passes, give your teeth a good brushing. Here are some other tips for keeping your teeth healthy while you're pregnant:

- ✔ Keep teeth clean particularly around the gum line.
- ✔ Brush with fluoride toothpaste three times (or more) a day when possible.
- ✔ Floss three times (or more) a day when possible.

Dental Visits During Pregnancy

As soon as you know that you are pregnant, visit your dentist for an overall evaluation of your teeth and gums and a good cleaning. At that time, the dentist or hygienist can give you special mouth care tips to use during your pregnancy.

- ◆ Continue regular dental visits throughout pregnancy.
- ◆ Avoid any elective treatment during the first three months of pregnancy.
- ◆ X-rays are *not* recommended. If an emergency makes x-rays necessary, be sure to wear the lead apron. If you have any questions concerning x-rays, consult immediately with your physician.

Sink Your Teeth into This: Most dental procedures can be done anytime during pregnancy, especially regularly scheduled hygiene appointments. We can't stress enough how important it is to keep teeth and gums clean. Consult your physician before having any dental procedure that requires anesthesia or medication.

The ABCs of a Child's "Healthy Teeth" Diet

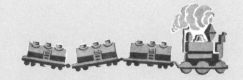

EATING FOR TWO

A baby's tooth buds begin to form between the fifth or sixth week of pregnancy. What you eat during this time nourishes the baby's development. Unless the doctor advises otherwise, expectant moms should eat a balanced diet with foods high in calcium and phosphorous — key building blocks for healthy baby's teeth.

BIRTH TO 2 YEARS

Sucking is an important part of facial muscle development, and it is important not to take the bottle away too early. But to avoid baby bottle tooth decay, don't give bottles at naps or bedtime. By the time the baby reaches the age of one, you may be weaning him or her off the bottle and encouraging your child to drink from a cup. As your child nears the magic age of two, he or she has been introduced to relatives, babysitters, and friends. In other words, what is put into the child's mouth is no longer totally influenced by Mom and Dad. Eating patterns and habits—good and not so good — are beginning to develop. Watch your child's "sweets" intake.

3 TO 6 YEARS

Eating habits that are formed during this period will have long-lasting consequences for your child's teeth. Don't let your toddler sip on soft drinks, suck on sweets, etc. When given a choice, children will usually choose the food that is high in sugar. Give them healthy snack food alternatives.

7 TO 12 YEARS

Now is the time when your early "good eating" training will come in handy. Kids' diets tend to take a dive at this age. Between snacks at their friends' homes and tempting TV commercials, it is close to impossible to monitor what they eat. Educate yourself and your children. Explain what foods are not healthy for teeth (acidic juice drinks and sodas, for example). Read labels and look at the sugar content. Every five grams of sugar equals one teaspoon of table sugar. That's eight to 10 teaspoons of sugar in each 12-ounce can of cola.

13 TO 18 YEARS

This is a tough age for any intervention from Mom and Dad. Many teenagers are drinking three to four sodas a day and have plenty of pocket change left over to load up on fast foods, donuts, and a variety of decay-producing snacks. Promote water and sugarless gum in place of sodas and sweets. Also, at this age teens are at risk for catching decay or gum disease from their friends. Explain this and caution them not to drink (or eat) from someone else's cup, bottle, or straw.

BIRTH TO 2 YEARS
The Fruits of Your Labor

*W*hen you take care of Mama's teeth you also take care of baby's teeth. Your newborn could be just a kiss away from catching your decay or gum infection. Remember decay and gum disease are transmissible. Without meaning to, you can spread bad bacteria to your newborn's mouth. We suggest that you make sure everyone in the family is in good oral health when your baby arrives.

What Happens After Baby Is Born?

After your baby is born and during its first year, all your time seems to be spent sitting in doctors' offices. Now we are asking you to add a dental visit to your growing list of "things to do." No one ever knows how much time and energy goes into taking care of a baby unless they have been through it before. We suggest that you begin your search for a pediatric dentist while you still have some time on your hands—before your due date.

Looking for "Dr. Tooth Guardian"

Decisions regarding your family's health care are important and require time and research. Choosing your child's dentist certainly falls into that category. We suggest you find a pediatric dentist in your area—a dental specialist who is uniquely trained to treat children from infancy through their teenage years.

Pediatric dentists make kids feel special and their offices are especially designed for children. It is our opinion that most general dentists do not have the extra time or training and staff to help young, apprehensive children feel good about seeing the dentist and taking care of their teeth. Certainly there are general dentists who fit the category of "Dr. Tooth Guardian," and your dentist is the first person you should turn to for a referral. Ask if he or she is comfortable working on children. If not, ask for a recommendation.

If it is necessary to continue your search, ask around for referrals from parents you know and trust. When you are asking for referrals, also ask what makes their child's dentist so special. Here are a few other sources for referrals:

- ✔ Family and friends
- ✔ Your children's school or daycare workers or other parents
- ✔ Co-workers
- ✔ Church members
- ✔ Your child's pediatrician

Time to Do Your Research

Once you have your referrals, it is time to act.

- ◆ Arrange for a short "get acquainted" visit with the dentist and staff. Most dental offices will let you do this before actually committing to an examination or treatment.

- ◆ Let your parental intuition kick in. During the on-site visit, determine if you and your child will feel comfortable. Is a long-term relationship possible with this dentist?

- ◆ Ask what techniques the dentist uses to calm and persuade a young child to cooperate with treatment. Does the dentist use medication or any type of physical restraint? It is important that you are comfortable with the dentist's reply. At one time, two restraining procedures—the hand-over-mouth restraint and the use of a papoose (similar to a straight jacket) were used in dental offices. In fact, dentists were *taught* to use these restraints in dental school. Of course, these practices are no longer appropriate (but may still be used by someone somewhere).

- ◆ Ask if anyone on the dental team is trained in children's CPR. (This is especially important if your child has asthma, drug allergies, or any condition which involves the heart and lungs).

WHAT IS A PEDIATRIC DENTIST?

A pediatric dentist (also called a *pedodontist)* receives two to three years of post-dental school training and specializes in comprehensive dental care for infants, children, and adolescents. The very young, pre-teens, and teenagers all need different approaches for dealing with their behavior, their dental growth and development, and future dental problems. The pediatric dentist is qualified to meet these needs. You can expect to find a dental practice where the staff is experienced and set up for working exclusively with kids.

Pediatric dentistry is all about trying to prevent problems. Only a small percentage of active dentists are trained as pediatric dental specialists, which means you may or may not be able to find one in your area. If you can't find a pediatric dentist in your area, look for a general dentist whose patient base includes a large percentage of kids of all ages.

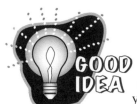

■ ■ ■ ■ ■ ■ ■ ■ ■

EIGHT STEPS TO A CHILD'S HEALTHY, HAPPY SMILE

Parental involvement is the key to a lifetime of good dental habits.

1. Dental and hygiene visits
2. Brushing
3. Flossing
4. Fluoride
5. Sealants
6. Sports safety
7. Healthy diet
8. Early orthodontic evaluation

■ ■ ■ ■ ■ ■ ■ ■ ■

When you go for a "get acquainted" visit, the dentist is also getting acquainted with you and your child and determining what he or she needs to do in order to make the child feel more comfortable. So don't be shy about arranging the "get acquainted" visit *prior* to making an actual appointment.

After You've Chosen Dr. Tooth Guardian

Once you've chosen a dentist for your child, it is better not to attempt to interfere with the communication between the dentist and child, unless the dentist or hygienist requests help. We know this will be hard for some parents, but try to remember that in every good doctor/patient relationship, trust is the key ingredient. *Your child is the patient* who is learning to trust the dentist.

Sink Your Teeth into This: If at all possible, try to avoid having your child's first appointment be an emergency appointment! Some dentists will refuse to perform any treatment when they have never met the child before. This is so important because the dentist and patient must build a trusting relationship *before* the dentist starts any "scary" procedures. If right off the bat, a child is given a shot, or his or her mouth is forced to remain open for a long time, or the dentist uses the drill and the sound frightens the child, he or she will surely grow up hating to go to the dentist.

Beware of Baby Bottle Tooth Decay!

Imagine this scenario: You are bringing three-year-old Amy to the hospital where she will be put under general anesthesia to have her decayed baby teeth protected and covered with silver (or white) crowns. Amy wakes up to a mouthful of silver teeth that may remain in place for another four to eight years. Eating is foreign and she grows up cruelly ridiculed by other children. Her self-esteem is shattered, and the scarring memory lingers for a lifetime.

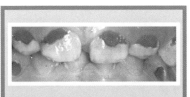

The tragic aftermath of baby bottle tooth decay.

Baby bottle tooth decay (also known as nursing decay) is caused by frequent and long exposures to liquids that contain sugar including: breast milk, formula, fruit juice, and other sweetened drinks.

As parents, we know how tempting it is to put a cranky baby to bed with a bottle of juice or milk to quiet them. But once you (and grandparents, uncles, aunts, and babysitters) grasp the trauma of baby bottle tooth decay, you will never want to expose your child to habits that can lead to this disabling destruction of primary teeth.

TEETHING TIPS

When baby teeth start pushing through the gums, teething symptoms may include restlessness, drooling, irritability, loss of appetite, or sporadic crying. It helps to keep baby's mouth clean. Use a damp rag and gently massage the gums. This will relieve some of the teething discomfort. Also try a chilled teething toy or teething gel.

Here's a tip for preventing baby bottle tooth decay. When putting baby to bed with a bottle for a nap or at night or for any prolonged time, use only water. Also, to prevent nursing decay, pediatric dentists recommend that a child be weaned from the breast by approximately 12 months of age.

Baby's Tooth Care

A new baby's mouth care should begin within the first few days after he or she is born. Plaque and bacteria will begin to collect on the baby's gums after every feeding. Get off to a good healthy start. Put your clean fingers in baby's mouth and massage the gums and cheeks. It's interesting that we feel comfortable putting our fingers in our children's ears, and wiping their eyes, nose, and lips (and everything else),

THE "KNEE TO KNEE" EXAM

GOOD IDEA

A new mom routinely turns to the pediatrician for all the answers about her baby's physical needs including the baby's mouth. But the pediatrician is not trained to examine your baby's dental needs. So it only makes sense to choose a dentist at the same time that you choose a pediatrician—right from the start. The dentist will monitor and watch over your child's oral health. When baby's first tooth comes in, pediatric dentist Gordon Strole does a visual exam on his tiny patients using an easy, "knee to knee" technique. It works like this: The baby lies on the parent's lap facing Mom (or Dad). The dentist sits on a stool and is knee to knee with the parent. Mom tilts the baby's head backward toward the dentist and holds the baby's hands while the dentist examines the child's mouth.

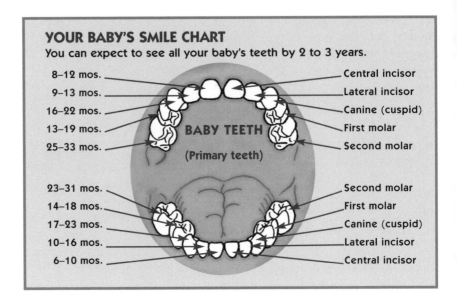

YOUR BABY'S SMILE CHART
You can expect to see all your baby's teeth by 2 to 3 years.

8–12 mos.	Central incisor
9–13 mos.	Lateral incisor
16–22 mos.	Canine (cuspid)
13–19 mos.	First molar
25–33 mos.	Second molar

BABY TEETH
(Primary teeth)

23–31 mos.	Second molar
14–18 mos.	First molar
17–23 mos.	Canine (cuspid)
10–16 mos.	Lateral incisor
6–10 mos.	Central incisor

but the physical act of putting our fingers into a baby's mouth seems foreign or forbidden. You have our blessing. And the more you do it, the more comfortable you and your baby will feel. In fact, you will discover that baby will use your fingers as a pacifier.

After each feeding and bedtime:

◆ Gently wipe baby's gums with a clean, soft, damp wash cloth or gauze to remove bacteria and plaque. This routine helps baby become accustomed to having someone's hands inside his or her mouth. The cleaning ritual also prepares the baby for the time when the first tooth "comes in" (or erupts).

After baby's first tooth emerges:

◆ Brush the tooth (or teeth) twice a day using water and a tiny, very soft bristle toothbrush designed for toddlers. Continue to wipe the baby's gums with a damp rag.

6 to 12 Months: The "Ideal" First Trip to the Dentist

The ideal first dental visit takes place when the baby is between the age of six months and one year, around the time when babies typically get their first tooth (see the primary teeth diagram shown above). Getting a dental exam at this age helps a child build a comfort level with the dentist. In fact, a book about overcoming the fear and loathing of dentists would have no audience if everyone started going at this tender age.

Preventing Early Dental Problems

There's that magic word again—prevention. The earlier the dental visit, the better the chance of preventing dental problems.

Dental concerns for very young children include:

- **Decay.** This is the time to prevent "baby bottle tooth decay."

- **Gum disease.** A child can show some mild inflammation of gum tissue as early as age two.

- **Fluoride.** The dentist will evaluate the fluoride in your child's diet and may recommend using supplements or reducing fluoride.

- **Hygiene.** The dentist or hygienist will give you age-specific brushing and mouth care tips and techniques.

A HAPPY BABY DENTAL VISIT

Practice risk-free dentistry for your children. Don't make your child's first dental visit an emergency. It's tough on everyone — baby, parents, and the dentist. Start your child's dental visits at an early age to:

- Avoid traumatic dental emergencies (excluding an accident).

- Avoid having your child put under anesthesia in order to do dental procedures.

- Keep your child's teeth healthy.

- Make dental procedures unnecessary.

- Protect your child from being afraid of going to the dentist.

The first appointment can be a happy baby visit. It should begin what can be a lifetime of favorable dental experiences. The first appointment also gives you a feel for whether the dentist is a good match for your child—prior to the time when any dental work may be necessary. If after the initial visit you are uncomfortable with the dentist or any of the dental team, continue your search.

WHAT'S THE FUSS? WHY BABY THOSE BABY TEETH?

Pediatric dentists will tell you the comment they hear most often from parents is, *"They are only baby teeth. They are going to fall out anyway. Why do we have to fix them?"*

Many parents don't consider baby teeth important because adult teeth eventually replace them. However, primary (baby) teeth play an important role in guiding adult teeth into position. The key is to make sure the baby teeth serve the child until the permanent teeth are all in place. That may be as long as 10 or 12 years—longer than some of us drive our cars.

Healthy baby teeth also play an important role in developing self-esteem and social skills. Decay, once started, can spread rapidly in children's teeth causing them to be extra-sensitive to hot and cold which, in turn, can affect the child's nutrition and/or disposition. When baby teeth must be pulled out because of decay, it can hinder the child's speech and his or her ability to swallow. Also, the space left for the permanent teeth may need to be recreated by orthodontics.

■ ■ ■ ■ ■ ■ ■ ■ ■ ■ ■

GETTING YOUR MONEY'S WORTH!

18 Years of Dental Prevention for a Lifetime of Smiles

Fill in the blanks with the costs of your child's cleaning and dental visits and you will get a good idea of the cost effectiveness of dental prevention.

• • • • • • • • • • • • • • • • • •

WHAT'S THE PRICE OF PREVENTION?

Based on two dental visits per year from age 1 to age 18:

17 years **X** 2 visits per year = 34 total

34 cleaning visits **X** $_____= $_____

17 doctors visits done at a hygiene appointment **X** $_____= $_____

TOTAL COST $_____

■ ■ ■ ■ ■ ■ ■ ■ ■ ■ ■

Age 2: The Next-Best First Trip to the Dentist

Because you want your child's dental visits to be pain-free and fun, the next-best time to bring baby to the dentist is at age two. At this age, thanks to your early home care prevention efforts, baby's teeth and gums should be decay and disease free.

Children between the ages of two and four who have never visited a dentist are at greater risk of having tooth decay and of developing a fear of going to the dentist.

When children get a bit older, they confuse going to the dentist with visits to their pediatrician. They remember painful immunization shots and become fearful that the dentist will hurt them too. So avoid using the phrase, *"We're going to see the doctor."*

DETECTING PROBLEMS

☒ **Thrush.** Oral thrush is a fungal infection (*Candida albicans*) in the mouth and common in infants and toddlers. If you are breast-feeding, thrush can be passed back and forth between mother and child. Symptoms for mom are nipples that are red, itchy or burning and shooting pains in the breast after feeding. Baby may have a diaper rash, white patches on the inside of his or her mouth and may be reluctant to nurse. If you suspect you or your baby have thrush, be sure to call your physician to get examined and treated.

☒ **Into the Mouths of Babes.**

Before age two, you don't need to worry about thumb-sucking. This is a natural reflex for infants. Sucking, after all, is one of the first functions a baby uses to eat. And how baby loves it when he or she manage to get a whole fist into his/her mouth. It helps to make baby feel happy and

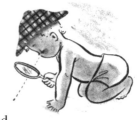

secure. As children grow older, they usually lose interest and their thumb-sucking tapers off. What about pacifiers? The use of a pacifier is only a problem if extended over a long time. Most children will stop both sucking their thumbs or using pacifiers on their own. But if they are still sucking something (fingers, thumbs, blanket, etc.) when permanent teeth arrive, discuss it with your child's dentist.

⊠ Epstein's Pearls. Here's something you *don't* need to worry about! It is a perfectly normal condition. A newborn baby has 20 primary teeth under the gums. A newborn's mouth also has a layer of tissue lining the bottom lip. The purpose of this tissue is to help the baby's mouth latch on to Mom's breast while nursing. These "suckling pads" may become swollen and hard or you may see little white dots inside the mouth on the gum pads. This is normal and doesn't require any type of dental or medical attention as the "pearls" are easily shed.

DOS AND DON'TS

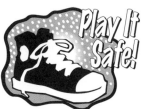

- ◆ *Do* limit juice drinks to 10% or less of the baby's daily diet. Juice encourages tooth decay.

- ◆ *Do* wipe baby's gums with a soft, damp cloth after each feeding.

- ◆ *Do* use either your finger or a small brush in the child's mouth twice a day when baby's first teeth "come in."

- ◆ *Do* discuss a fluoride supplement with your child's dentist if you live in an area with low fluoride content. Fluoride strengthens the tooth's enamel.

- ◆ *Don't* give your child any fluoride if he or she is under six months of age. If you have any questions or doubts, discuss it with your child's dentist and pediatrician.

- ◆ *Do* be careful when adding water to formula because it may exceed recommended levels of fluoride. It is better to use distilled water, purified water, or tap water filtered with a reverse osmosis filter. Too much fluoride in the diet will show up later as white spots on the permanent teeth (fluorosis). On the other hand. . .

- ◆ *Don't* use only bottled water (which in most cases has no fluoride) or you may get too little fluoride in the diet. Consult with your child's dentist and pediatrician.

If Only
I Knew Then
What I Know Now...

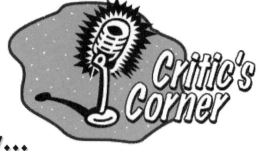

*W*e asked parents to share their thoughts about our recommendation that baby's dental care begin shortly after birth and that their trip to the dentist occur as soon as the first baby tooth emerges. Wow! Did we get reactions:

- ◆ Parents with more than two children shouted and groaned, *"Get real! We don't have time to go to one more doctor's appointment or spend time wiping baby's gums after every feeding. We're busy getting kids ready for school, driving to soccer games, running after toddlers, and taking care of a newborn."*

- ◆ A few parents even shot back, *"You're just trying to get parents to spend more money on the dentist."*

Then there are parents like me who feel guilty about not starting their children's prevention and care at a younger age. I asked a friend (who happens to be a top-notch dentist) if he and his wife were wiping their four-month-old baby's gums after each feeding. He looked at me with genuine surprise and said no. That's when I realized that if this professional insider didn't know (or didn't feel compelled to practice) early prevention with his child, regular parents like you and me will find it tough to make the time and take the effort.

So forgive us for giving what, at times, must seem like unreasonable advice. What we are trying to do is break through old norms. But think about this. The time when your baby's teeth are untouched by any dental disease is your one chance to protect something (and someone) *perfect.*

Consider our advice as a set of "personal best practices." Some may not be practical for you and your family's lifestyle. But at least now you know how high the moon and what star to shoot for.

3 TO 6 YEARS
The Growing Years

*A*t age three, kids start to have minds of their own. Usually by this age, they have firm opinions about doctor visits and what foods they will eat. If the child has been to the dentist prior to this age, he or she should have no fear or frustration about dental appointments. On the other hand, if at this age he or she is going to the dentist for the first time, the situation may not be as easy. Anything the child hasn't already been trained to do (such as potty training, going to bed on time, or taking medicine) takes a lot of extra effort from parents. And now you can add going to the dentist to that list.

By age six, your child's jaws are growing to make room for the permanent teeth. The first permanent molars usually

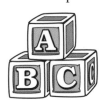

erupt between ages five and six. Parents often mistake them for baby teeth. These molars are especially important because they help determine the shape of the lower face. They also affect the position and health of permanent teeth. It is hard to

---

SEALANTS: ONE DECAY BARRIER

A sealant is a clear plastic material that protects tooth surfaces that have deep grooves and pits. Often these surfaces include the chewing surfaces of back teeth, which is where most cavities in children are found. Properly applied sealants create a barrier against decay. But this doesn't mean you can get lax about cleaning the teeth. Children still need to brush at least twice a day and floss *between* their teeth daily.

Sealants are only one step in preventing decay and they don't seal between the teeth. Ice or hard candy can chip or break the sealant and acidic-type beverages can eat away at the protective sealant cover. Don't be surprised if sealants need to be replaced. Your child's dentist may or may not suggest sealants as the treatment of choice. Instead, the dentist may put a filling material over the grooves to keep out plaque and food to decrease the risk of tooth decay.

■ ■ ■ ■ ■ ■ ■ ■ ■

HOW MUCH FLUORIDE?

Don't use excessive amounts of fluoride because it can cause white spots (*fluorosis*) in permanent teeth. When this happens, the enamel formation gets disrupted and causes cosmetic changes to the teeth that make them look chalky white.

To find out the level of fluoride in your local drinking water call your local water company and ask, "What concentration of fluoride is in your 'finished' drinking water?" The EPA recommends that the maximum amount of fluoride is 0.7 to 1.0 milligrams per liter. Most bottled water does not contain fluoride. Therefore, some children may be getting too little fluoride, and the dentist (or pediatrician) may recommend a fluoride supplement.

■ ■ ■ ■ ■ ■ ■ ■ ■ ■ ■ ■

imagine, but those little six-year molars will be in baby's mouth for another 70-plus years. So treat them kindly!

Toddler's Tooth Care

Once a child has most of his or her baby teeth, it is time for you to start flossing them. Brush at least twice daily and always at bedtime. Make your brushing routine fun and the child will look forward to it. Be creative. Begin a ritual of singing a song, listening to the child's favorite music, or making up a story about the "brushing and flossing fairy." Let the child begin brushing; then finish for him or her.

You might notice that your child has spaces between the teeth. No need to worry. This is common because the permanent teeth can be twice as large as the teeth they are replacing. Flossing at this point is mainly to get the child in the habit of seeing and feeling floss in his/her mouth.

Six Things to Remember about Toddler Tooth Care:

1. Use a soft, small toothbrush.
2. Use only a pea-sized amount of toothpaste.
3. Don't let children eat toothpaste.
4. Always brush before bedtime.
5. Be a positive role model. Let your kids see you brush and floss your teeth.
6. Don't share your toothbrush with your kids.

DETECTING TODDLER PROBLEMS

Watch for CLUES

❌ **Into the Mouths of Babes**. If your child's thumb sucking persists at age four, it may be time for concern. The dentist should evaluate the situation. If any damage or malformation is present in the mouth, the dentist may recommend a special retainer to inhibit sucking.

❌ **A Tooth in Crisis**. Between the ages of three and six, kids fall a lot, often hitting their mouths while riding bikes and playing. At this age, gum tissue heals quickly. Baby teeth can be hit, banged, or chipped and the injury won't necessarily have any effect on the permanent teeth. As a precaution though, always call the dentist as soon as possible if you have any concerns.

DOS AND DON'TS

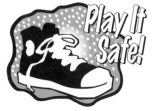

- ◆ **Do** replace your child's toothbrush every one to two months and immediately following a cold or the flu.

- ◆ **Do** have your child brush at least twice a day.

- ◆ **Don't** let your child go to bed without brushing.

- ◆ **Don't** let your child drink juice, milk, or soft drinks during the night either by cup or by bottle.

- ◆ **Do** keep toothpaste out of the reach of children. If ingested in excess, it can cause the child to become ill.

- ◆ **Do** store toothbrushes so they do not touch each other.

- ◆ **Don't** share toothbrushes.

- ◆ **Don't** attempt to re-insert a baby tooth into baby's mouth if it is knocked out or dislodged. Call your dentist immediately.

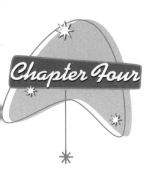

Chapter Four

7 TO 12 YEARS
The Tooth Fairy Years

*N*ow is the time to introduce the "Tooth Fairy," because baby teeth are falling out and permanent teeth are growing in. What a thrilling passage for parents and child when those baby teeth are gone. We celebrate the tooth's demise with toys and money secretly placed under the child's pillow in the name of the "Tooth Fairy."

Meanwhile, the permanent teeth come in without fanfare. From the start, permanent teeth are taken for granted even though they will be expected to perform for many decades. We often hear parents saying, *"I don't see how my child's mouth is going to hold those big teeth. They look so much big-*

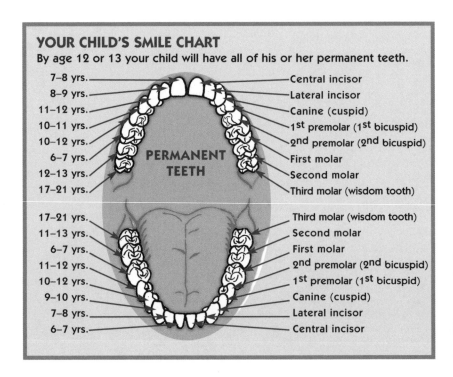

YOUR CHILD'S SMILE CHART
By age 12 or 13 your child will have all of his or her permanent teeth.

7–8 yrs.	Central incisor
8–9 yrs.	Lateral incisor
11–12 yrs.	Canine (cuspid)
10–11 yrs.	1st premolar (1st bicuspid)
10–12 yrs.	2nd premolar (2nd bicuspid)
6–7 yrs.	First molar
12–13 yrs.	Second molar
17–21 yrs.	Third molar (wisdom tooth)
17–21 yrs.	Third molar (wisdom tooth)
11–13 yrs.	Second molar
6–7 yrs.	First molar
11–12 yrs.	2nd premolar (2nd bicuspid)
10–12 yrs.	1st premolar (1st bicuspid)
9–10 yrs.	Canine (cuspid)
7–8 yrs.	Lateral incisor
6–7 yrs.	Central incisor

PERMANENT TEETH

ger than the baby teeth." This is that awkward, "ugly ducking" stage that all kids must pass through.

At this stage, kids' schedules pick up after school with activities and sports. Weekday mornings get rushed and hectic for families and the bathrooms are a busy place. In response to *"Did you brush your teeth?"* kids reply, *"Mom, I'm late. I don't have time to brush."*

What can you do? The best answer is to get your children up 10 minutes earlier and make them brush.

But our "get real" answer is:

♦ Set a firm time for brushing before bedtime.

♦ No skipping allowed.

♦ If your kids brush every night, skipping the morning once in awhile will not jeopardize their oral health.

WARNING SIGNS OF POTENTIAL DECAY

When the child starts brushing on his or her own, it's a good idea to see how well he or she is doing. You may need to tag team and let your child begin the brushing, while you do the finish work. If you notice that food stays caught in the pits and grooves of your child's teeth after brushing on his/her own, either the child is not brushing thoroughly or the grooves in the teeth are very deep. Discuss this with the dentist. Some treatment options include:

♦ Cleaning out the grooves and making sure there is no decay. If no decay is present, the dentist can seal the area with a sealant.

♦ If there is decay, the dentist will put in a stronger filling material.

Your Child's Tooth Care

By now your child is probably able to brush his or her teeth on his/her own. But you will still need to supervise to make sure he or she is doing a thorough job. Ask the dentist or hygienist if your child is ready to use an electric toothbrush. It shows your support and rewards the child for doing such a good job with tooth care.

Anytime your child's mouth is not clean, it becomes a potential site for decay or gum disease. If your child has gingivitis (infection of the gums) you may see puffy gums and notice a little blood the first few times that you floss his or her teeth. With daily flossing, the gums will get healthier and the bleeding will stop. If the problem persists, call your dentist. By the time your child is nine or 10, he or she should be able to floss on his/her own.

Involve your child in the flossing process:

♦ Position yourself so you can see your child's teeth. It's easiest to work from behind with your child's head tilted backward toward you.

- ◆ Let the child hold a hand mirror to observe the flossing process to see how it's done.

- ◆ It only makes sense that if it hurts to floss, kids won't do it. So floss gently, hugging the tooth, sliding the floss up and down and under the gum. Avoid cutting into the gums with the floss.

Sink Your Teeth into This: Around age 12, when boys and girls start to get sweet on each other, children worry about bad breath. Tell them that brushing their tongue will help. Or buy a tongue scraper. If the bad breath persists, consult your dentist or hygienist for an evaluation. It may be due to allergies or post-nasal drip.

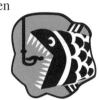

When Your Child Needs Calming at the Dentist

If your child's first visit to the dentist is between the ages of seven and 12, you may have to drag the child to the appointment kicking and screaming. And more than likely, some type of dental treatment will be necessary. If the child needs calming, the doctor may suggest using a calming agent like nitrous oxide (often referred to as nitrous) to perform the dental procedure.

What Is Nitrous Oxide/Oxygen?

Nitrous oxide is perhaps the safest calming agent in dentistry. It is commonly used when a child feels anxious during treatment. It doesn't knock the child out, but makes the child feel silly and relaxed while fully conscious. Nitrous is usually accepted easily by children and is quickly eliminated by the body. Nitrous oxide should be administered to your child only

---

WHEN KIDS PLAY SPORTS

The National Youth Sports Foundation for the Prevention of Athletic Injuries reports that dental injuries are the most common type of oro-facial injury sustained while playing sports. A mouth guard acts as a cushion to the blow of an injury and distributes pressure throughout the entire jaw. Mouth guards protect more than broken teeth. They also help to prevent broken jaws, concussions, cerebral hemorrhages, and neck injuries. Two types of mouth guards that are frequently recommended are the custom-made or the "boil and bite." Your dentist can custom-make a mouth guard or you can choose the "boil and bite" mouth guard from a sporting goods store. Whatever type of mouth guard your child wears, it should fit well and the child should be able to speak and breathe comfortably while wearing it.

with your permission and only when necessary. Sometimes the levels of nitrous oxide can be too heavy for a child, and the child may become temporarily nauseated and vomit. If you know ahead of time that nitrous will be administered, give your child little or no food before the dental visit.

Before Your Child Is Given Nitrous Oxide:

1. Review the child's medical history with the dentist.
2. Explain any respiratory condition that makes breathing through the nose difficult. It may limit the effectiveness of the nitrous.
3. Tell your dentist if your child is taking any medication on the day of the appointment.

Questions to Ask the Dentist and the Dental Team:

◆ What certificates and training does the dentist have to administer nitrous oxide?

◆ How many times has he or she administered sedation during similar dental procedures? What was the outcome of those procedures?

◆ What are the certification laws in the state for the use of nitrous oxide?

◆ Does the staff member who is monitoring (and/or administering) the nitrous oxide have the necessary certification?

There is nothing wrong with the doctor being put on alert. Good Dr. Tooth Guardians will welcome these questions. If the dentist seems uncomfortable with your questions or in any way reacts defensively, you can always seek another dentist.

When Anesthesia Is Necessary

Children who are afraid of the dentist or have been hurt by a dental procedure in the past and require extensive dental work can be impossible to work on while they are conscious. In order to perform the necessary treatment, there are times when a child must be heavily sedated. But parents must be cautioned that children have died from over-sedation in dental offices due to inexperience, lack of training, and/or an office not fully equipped to deal with emergencies.

Children are not tiny adults. When extensive dental work requires deep or heavy sedation, the child should be under the direct supervision of a qualified pediatric dentist and pediatric anesthesiologist.

Questions to Ask Before a Child Is Sedated:

- Is the anesthesia or sedation absolutely necessary?

- What is the dentist's training for administering this procedure?

- Who will be monitoring the child while the dentist is doing the dentistry? And what is their training?

- On how many patients has the doctor administered this medication, sedation, or anesthesia?

- What was the outcome?

- Are there any side effects?

- How will the dentist handle an emergency, if something goes wrong?

DETECTING OTHER DENTAL PROBLEMS

☒ **Smokeless Tobacco.** The National Cancer Society reports that over 12 million people use some form of smokeless tobacco and the largest increase over the last decade has been among the 8-year-olds to 17-year-olds. The health consequences of tobacco use include decay, gum disease, and oral cancer. Talk to your kids about steering clear of smokeless tobacco.

☒ **Juvenile Periodontitis.** Usually first detected between ages 10 and 15, this rare but very serious gum disease can rapidly destroy bone around the front permanent teeth and around the first permanent molars. Check your child for signs of puffy gums, blood on the toothbrush, and complaints of tender, sore gums. If your child is getting regular, six-month dental check-ups, juvenile periodontitis will more than likely be discovered during an exam.

☒ **A Tooth in Crisis.** Accidents and athletic injuries may cause damage to the teeth and gums. If a tooth is chipped or broken, save the pieces and see your dentist immediately. If the tooth gets knocked out, pick it up by the crown. Never handle the roots. If the tooth is dirty, rinse *gently* in slow, running water. Don't scrub the tooth. Gently place the tooth back into the socket until you can get to the dentist's office. If this doesn't work, the tooth will have to either be stored in cold, whole milk or placed between your child's gum and cheek until you get to the dentist. If it is a baby tooth, do *not* re-insert it. Quick action can save a tooth that has been knocked completely out of the socket.

PLAY IT SAFE

◆ ***Don't*** assume that your child is doing an excellent job cleaning his or her teeth.

◆ ***Do*** check your child's teeth after the brushing routine.

◆ ***Do*** have your child wear a mouth guard for all contact sports (if possible for other sports activities, too).

◆ ***Do*** continue to check your child's teeth regularly to see if he or she is brushing correctly.

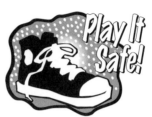

◆ ***Do*** examine your child's gums for any sign of gum disease such as red, puffy, and bleeding gums.

◆ ***Do*** check to see if your child's teeth are starting to be crowded. At your child's next dental visit, inquire about seeing an orthodontist for an evaluation.

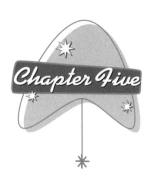

Chapter Five

13 TO 18 YEARS
Invasion of the Hormones

*A*lthough not yet adults, teens can lose their teeth in the same way that Mom and Dad can—only with more youthful vigor. But even though teens have all their permanent teeth just like adults, below the gum line is a different story. Teen teeth are trapped in a *JAWS 3* horror movie and are in danger of being eaten by runaway decay. A small area of decay in an adult can take years to spread. The same amount of decay in a teen will advance rapidly because the nerves in teen teeth are extremely large and more easily infected.

Lifestyle habits play a large role in how a teenager's teeth survive during this time of rampant decay. The teen years are a critical period for any person's teeth.

Teens' Tooth Care

It's a fact. After-school jobs, sports, homework, and activities with friends take a lot of your teenager's time. As schedules get stretched, teens delegate time spent on brushing and flossing according to their priorities. And taking care of their teeth falls low on the list.

During these years, parents run into resistance from their teenagers on all fronts. Brushing their teeth is no exception. The *"you gotta brush"* message starts to sound like a broken record, and no parent enjoys the job of nagging. Some parents feel that at this age they are violating their children's rights when asking them to brush. Many parents say their requests are falling on deaf ears. Be persistent. It *does* make a difference.

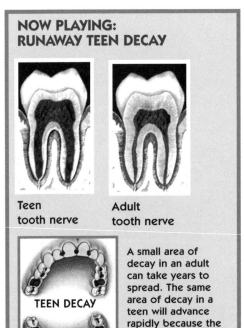

**NOW PLAYING:
RUNAWAY TEEN DECAY**

Teen
tooth nerve

Adult
tooth nerve

TEEN DECAY

A small area of decay in an adult can take years to spread. The same area of decay in a teen will advance rapidly because the nerves in teen teeth are extremely large and easily infected.

CALL!

One phone call will help take the heat off of Mom and Dad. Call to make a special hygiene appointment for your busy teen and let the hygienist do the talking.

A good hygienist can impress on your teenager that age, lifestyle, fluctuating hormones, and large tooth nerves make him or her highly susceptible to decay. Let the pros explain how brushing permanent teeth is different than caring for baby teeth. Unlike baby teeth, the larger and more crowded permanent teeth are much harder to keep clean. And gum tissue gets puffy and red and needs extra flossing.

When you call the dental office, explain the mouth care challenges you are facing with your teenager. Ask if the hygienist can tailor the visit to fit your teen's situation. The hygienist will give your teen practical, age-specific advice including:

TEEN TEETH NEED TOUGH LOVE

◆ A teen's decay advances more quickly because of the large tooth nerves.

◆ Teen lifestyle habits differ from adult's habits. For example, teens may eat more snacks, drink more sodas, have their tongues pierced, be more lax on mouth care, etc.

◆ The wisdom teeth (third molars) begin to come in.

◆ Braces need special cleaning.

◆ Teens often don't brush and floss as frequently and thoroughly as necessary.

◆ Flossing and brushing shortcuts for busy teens. (If your teen isn't flossing yet, it's tough to get him or her started. Let a pro handle this. It may take several cleaning visits before your teen really gets the hang of it.)

◆ Brushing and flossing tips unique to teen teeth. Teens in a hurry will quickly brush their back teeth and give their front teeth one quick swipe with the brush (or none). The hygienist can spot any brushing problems.

◆ Answers to concerns about bad breath. The hygienist can show your teen how to use a tongue scraper.

Ask the dentist or hygienist about brightening your teen's teeth with bleaching. This is a treat (especially after braces are removed) and a good incentive to get your teen to brush and floss more often.

GOOD IDEA

Make It Easy for Teens to Care for Their Teeth

◆ Supply plenty of "take along" floss, toothpaste, and extra toothbrushes for backpacks and lockers, as well as at home. Your teen may be surprised to learn he or she can brush somewhere other than home.

- Buy your teen an electric toothbrush.

- Breath-conscious teens often, without thinking, pop in sugary mints or candy to "sweeten" their breath. If your teen has a persistent breath problem, ask the dentist for help.

- When not able to brush after a meal, encourage your teen to rinse his or her mouth with water and/or chew a piece of sugarless gum. Keep plenty of water and sugarless gum available.

Sink Your Teeth into This: Many teens drive themselves to their dental appointments. As a result, two problems frequently occur. They skip the appointment, and/or when an important dental decision must be made, parents are not available for consultation. The best-case scenario is for parents to accompany the teen to the dentist. Be involved and stay informed. If you can't make it in person, get a report from the dentist or ask someone on the dental team to call you. Remember, any decisions made concerning your teenager's teeth will extend for the life of the teeth.

Wise Guidance for Wisdom Teeth

Wisdom teeth usually appear between the ages of 17 and 22. Your dentist can track the development of your teen's wisdom teeth using panoramic x-rays. If your teen is getting regular dental exams, the dentist will be monitoring the wisdom teeth and will know when it is necessary to surgically remove them. By the way, removal is *not* always recommended.

BE SMART ABOUT WISDOM TEETH

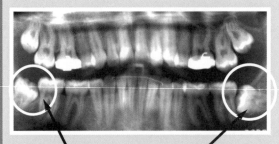

The panoramic image shows serious problems with the wisdom teeth. All four wisdom teeth will not erupt correctly. They cannot be properly cleaned. This can lead to decay of the adjacent teeth or gum disease. Find out when it is important to remove wisdom teeth or when you should leave them alone.

Wisdom Teeth Must Be Removed If:

- There are signs of serious infection.

- The areas around the teeth are tough to keep clean.

- There is pain and swelling.

- Partially erupted wisdom teeth crowd other teeth.

- Teeth cannot fully erupt because there is no room in the mouth.

DETECTING TEEN TOOTH PROBLEMS

Watch for CLUES

☒ **The Six-year Molars.** Parents must be watchful. There's no "small decay" in a teen's six-year molars because the nerves are so large. The treatment for extensive decay is root canal with a crown or extraction.

☒ **Decay Prone.** If your child is decay-prone, you have to ask yourself why. Your best bet may be to get a saliva test done to determine whether your teen has an overgrowth of the bacteria that causes decay.

☒ **Canker Sores.** These can be very unpleasant and often untimely, arriving right before a special date or prom night. They can be triggered by stress, certain foods (chocolate, acidic foods, or hard, rough food, for example) or due to some type of injury to the mouth.

☒ **Cold Sores.** These fever blisters can be triggered by fever, physical or emotional stress, or excessive exposure to the sun. There are ways to boost the immune system. And drinking eight glasses of water a day and eating wholesome foods will hasten the healing process. There are also anti-viral treatments for fever blisters that your dentist can prescribe. Oral medication and topical ointments are available. The dentist can determine the proper prescription.

☒ **Bulimia.** If your teenager has been diagnosed with bulimia, the next appointment you need to schedule is with the dentist. Stomach acid from frequent vomiting can be toxic to teeth and can lead to severe erosion of the enamel. Your dentist can diagnose bulimia (and in some cases, the dentist may be the first to spot the condition) and recommend treatment for the deteriorating tooth enamel. However, only a physician and/or psychologist can treat the actual eating disorder.

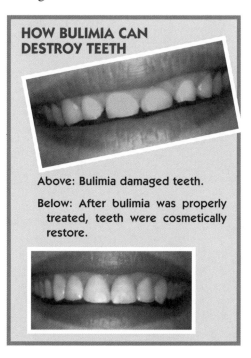

HOW BULIMIA CAN DESTROY TEETH

Above: Bulimia damaged teeth.

Below: After bulimia was properly treated, teeth were cosmetically restore.

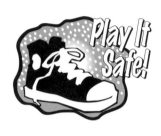

⊠ Piercing. Tongue piercing and lip piercing are becoming fairly common among today's teens. Reported complications of tongue piercing include chipped and damaged teeth, gum injury, prolonged bleeding, numbness, loss of taste, and interference with speech. Harboring food and bacteria, the metal stud becomes a cleaning challenge.

PLAY IT SAFE

◆ *Do* be watchful for decay and gum disease because teens are so susceptible. Dental check-ups every six months, diligent mouth care, and a good diet will be a tremendous help.

◆ *Do* set an example for your teenagers. Go to your regular dental check-ups and do your daily mouth care routine.

◆ *Do* check to make sure that your teenager shows up for his or her regular cleaning and/or dental and orthodontic appointments.

◆ *Do* keep in touch with your teen's dentist and dental team. Stay involved with your teen's dental care.

◆ *Don't* stock the refrigerator with sodas and ice cream

or have candy and sweets readily available.

◆ *Do* encourage mouth guards for your active teenagers.

◆ *Do* get rid of toothbrushes every one or two months, or sooner if frayed.

◆ *Do* stock up on dental floss.

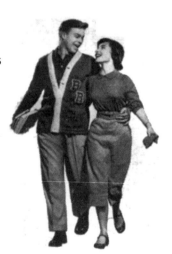

WILL MY CHILD NEED BRACES?

*T*hree dental questions foremost in most parents' minds are:

- Does my child have cavities?
- Is my child brushing her/his teeth correctly?
- Do you think he or she will need braces?

Of course there is no such thing as a typical child, but there are children who typically will need an early orthodontic exam. The only hard and fast rule that applies to kids and braces is that when braces are indicated, the best time to get an orthodontic exam is between the ages of five and seven. This is an age-specific *"window of opportunity."* For some children, early treatment achieves results that are possible only when the face and jaw is still growing.

How will you know if early treatment is necessary? It depends on the child. This is why regular dental and hygiene check-ups are so important. Children are in a constant flux of change and growth. When children start losing baby teeth and begin getting permanent teeth, parents usually notice if the teeth are growing in

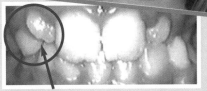

EARLY EVALUATION DETECTS CROSS BITE

This eight-year-old has four permanent front teeth. The rest are baby teeth. Photo "A" shows that her upper teeth are incorrectly positioned behind her lower teeth. This is a cross bite. She will wear an expander, and eventually braces, to correct the cross bite and to make room for her front permanent teeth.

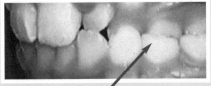

A SIDE VIEW — Notice her cross bite.

B Notice crowding of this front permanent tooth.

■ ■ ■ ■ ■ ■ ■ ■ ■ ■ ■

BRACE YOURSELF

When teeth and jaws do not fit and work together properly the condition is called "malocclusion" (also referred to as a "bad bite"). This occurs because:

◆ Teeth are crooked.

◆ Teeth are overcrowded.

◆ Teeth are out of alignment.

◆ Jaws don't meet properly.

More than likely, braces will be the treatment of choice. A "bad bite" becomes noticeable between the ages of five and 12 when permanent teeth are emerging.

■ ■ ■ ■ ■ ■ ■ ■ ■ ■ ■

crooked. General dentists and pediatric dentists are trained to spot potential problems during the child's periodic cleanings and check-ups. If the dentist has any concerns, he or she should address these concerns with you or refer your child to an orthodontist or a dentist trained in orthodontics. It is important to learn as much as you can about your child's condition and to ask questions. Remember, early detection means less trauma, less expense, and better results in the long run.

More than Just Straight Teeth

We all understand that braces reposition teeth and the rewards are obvious— straighter teeth, a beautiful and healthy smile, and a boost to the child's self esteem. What is not so obvious is that braces can also reconstruct facial structure. Skeletal problems such as protruding teeth, cross bites, overbites, or jaws that are underdeveloped can be significantly altered with braces to improve and change facial appearance. The time to get a child's adult face correctly positioned is at a younger age during the growing stage.

The Benefits of Braces

When teeth are crooked or crowded or sticking out ("buck teeth"), a child can be subjected to unfortunate nicknames and playground teasing. Other problems caused by crooked or crowded teeth include:

■ ■ ■ ■ ■ ■ ■ ■ ■ ■ ■

REMEMBER GRANDDAD HAD "BUCK TEETH!"

Some orthodontic problems are passed down from generation to generation. So your family tree may have something to do with your teeth, but you can also acquire problems on your own. However, If you know of any orthodontic problems in your family tree, bring them to the attention of your child's dentist.

■ ■ ■ ■ ■ ■ ■ ■ ■ ■ ■

◆ Higher risk of decay and gum disease due to difficulty cleaning crooked or crowded teeth.

◆ Protruding teeth that can be more easily chipped or fractured.

◆ Speech impediments caused by teeth not fitting together properly.

◆ Abnormal wear on tooth surfaces.

◆ Excessive stress on supporting bone and gum tissue.

◆ Misalignment of jaw joints resulting in headaches or facial or neck pain.

◆ Interference with proper jaw development.

The All-Important Diagnostic Records Exam

When a decision is made to begin early treatment, the proper diagnostic records are taken by the orthodontist (or pediatric dentist or general dentist).

These records should include:

1. A lateral head x-ray
2. A panoramic x-ray
3. A frontal head x-ray
4. A photograph of the face and teeth
5. Plaster models of the teeth
6. A comprehensive dental exam

With the exception of simple treatments such as a space maintainer for minor tooth movement, these records are *a must* when it is determined that your child needs braces.

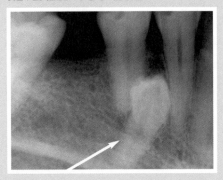

HIDDEN TOOTH REVEALED TOO LATE

If this patient had been given a comprehensive exam when younger, an orthodontist could have easily moved this impacted tooth into the correct position. This illustrates the value of a complete exam for early detection of problems.

The examination represents the standard of care in orthodontics regardless if you choose a general dentist, pediatric dentist, or an orthodontic specialist to treat your child for braces. You should *walk the other way* if the diagnostic records are not used as part of your child's orthodontic treatment plan.

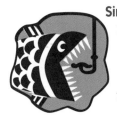

Sink Your Teeth into This: Regular visits to the family dentist must continue during orthodontic treatment. Good dental care and oral hygiene is essential. One of the biggest challenges for your child while wearing braces is keeping the teeth and gums clean and healthy.

LET'S GET SOMETHING STRAIGHT ABOUT ORTHODONTISTS

Orthodontics is the branch of dentistry that specializes in the diagnosis, prevention, and treatment of dental and facial irregularities. Orthodontic specialists practice orthodontics and dento-facial orthopedics.

What makes an orthodontist? Following dental school, orthodontists have completed an advanced education program and learned the special skills required to manage tooth movement and guide facial development. That's the technical answer. We like to say that an orthodontist provides a special treatment that brings teeth, lips, jaw, and face into harmony. In doing so, the orthodontist gives children (and adults) an opportunity to look good and feel their best.

A Calendar of Dental Visits

Children, like adults, need to be checked by the dentist twice a year. Tooth decay is not the only reason for going to see a dentist. The first and most important reason is prevention.

A Don't discuss your own dental experience with your child. Your child's dental visit will bear very little resemblance to your childhood visits. Be positive and upbeat.

B Don't use the phrase, *"We're going to see the doctor"* (the place where they get shots).

C If your child is two or older, bring him/her along with you to your next dental check-up. Often the dentist will allow the child to sit in the chair and get his/her teeth counted. It makes the child feel grown-up, and that makes it fun.

6 MONTHS TO 2 YEARS

At the first visit you will be asked to fill out your child's health history. If anything changes in the future, always let the dental team know.

Your dentist will do a visual exam to:

A Evaluate the gums and tissue inside the mouth.

B Inspect for signs of healthy tooth eruption.

C Check the child's jaw for normal development.

3 TO 6 YEARS

At this age, the dentist will monitor the baby teeth and may recommend sealants. During the exam, the dentist will provide an ongoing assessment of changes in the child's oral health and will:

A Review the child's medical and dental state of health.

B Check for dietary changes.

C Examine the need for fluoride or sealants.

D Clean the child's teeth.

E Take x-rays or digital images if necessary to check for decay between the teeth.

F Take a panoramic x-ray to determine if all permanent teeth are present and erupting properly and to check for any deformities, abscesses, or cysts.*

7 TO 12 YEARS

During this visit the dentist will:

A Take the first round of x-rays to check for decay between the teeth.

B Do a visual check for tooth decay.

C Check to see if the teeth fit together properly.

D Determine whether an orthodontic evaluation is necessary.

E Discuss replacing worn sealants.

F Clean and polish the teeth.

Be sure to ask to see the images and the orthodontic evaluation.

13 TO 18 YEARS

Any decisions made concerning the permanent teeth will last for the life of the tooth. Once a year, teenagers should receive a periodic dental exam which includes:

A Appropriate x-rays or digital images.

B A bite check to see how teeth fit together.

C An oral cancer screening.

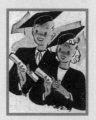

D A panoramic x-ray to check for developing wisdom teeth.

Your teen should be scheduled for cleanings at least every six months.

* PARENTS' NOTE: X-rays or digital images are only taken when they are necessary to diagnose tooth decay or abnormalities or for orthodontic problems. The frequency of x-rays depends on your child's individual needs. Your dentist should discuss your child's needs with you *before* any images are taken. High-speed film and proper shielding will make the amount of radiation exposure minimal. Digital imagery is a new technique for taking x-rays and offers 90% less radiation. A panoramic x-ray may be taken as early as age four or five to assess the development of permanent teeth.

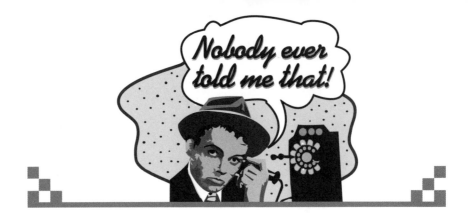

- During pregnancy women need frequent, preventive dental appointments to make sure they have no gum disease that may affect the fetus.

- If you start your baby's mouth care early and practice dental prevention, you will save a lot of money in the long run.

- Within a few days of a baby's birth, parents need to clean the baby's mouth, cheeks, and gums after feedings with a soft, damp piece of gauze or cloth. This is true for children of both nursing and non-nursing moms.

- Monitoring the health of your child's teeth and gums is outside the pediatrician's area of expertise. Dental diagnosis and treatment requires a pediatric dentist or general dentist.

- Between six and 12 months when the baby's first tooth comes in is the ideal time for your first dental visit with your baby.

- Even baby teeth may need orthodontic treatment. That's why it is so important to take your child to the dentist for regular check-ups.

- Not all bottled water contains fluoride. If you are relying on fluoride to supplement your child's dental needs, don't guess. Ask your dentist instead.

- If your child has a mouth injury, you may be able to save the tooth. Bring the tooth immediately (whole or in pieces) to the dentist. Be careful not to touch the root.

- Begin flossing your child's teeth at an early age as soon as he or she gets a few baby teeth in. This will get your child used to the process.

- If necessary, your child's jaw structure can be altered by orthodontics. This is best done when "a window of opportunity " exists for changing facial structure.

- The older a person is, the more difficult it will be to remove wisdom teeth and the longer it will take to heal.

- Your child's toothbrush needs to be replaced every one to two months. This is especially important after an illness.

- To prevent baby bottle tooth decay, don't put baby to bed with milk or juice in a bottle.

- Parents have the option of having a qualified pediatric anesthesiologist present if a child needs to be sedated in order to do necessary dental work.

- When permanent molars emerge, have the dentist or hygienist check to see if sealants or some type of coverage will be necessary to help prevent decay.

- Children can get advanced gum disease at an early age. This is rare, but it happens. It is called juvenile periodontitis.

- Even inherited physical appearances such as buck teeth can sometimes be corrected by orthodontia.

- Children need only a small pea-sized amount of toothpaste on their toothbrushes. Don't let them eat toothpaste because they may ingest too much fluoride.

- Parents should start early putting their fingers in their baby's mouth to clean it and to get the baby used to the feeling of having the teeth wiped and brushed.

- Remember that your child's permanent teeth will be performing in his or her mouth for 70 years or more!

SECTION V:

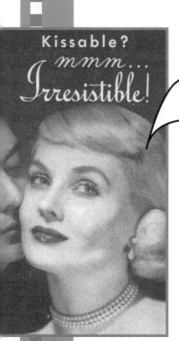

RESTORING YOUR MOUTH:
Teeth That Fit, Function, Feel Good, and Look Great!

Kissable? mmm... Irresistible!

The investment I made in my teeth is paying off!

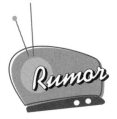

Rumor At my age, I'm too old to be investing money in my teeth.

The older you get, the more important your teeth are to your health. Aging can also make it harder to adjust to change. Losing your teeth causes huge changes in the way you chew, speak, eat, and digest your food.

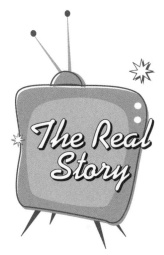

The Real Story

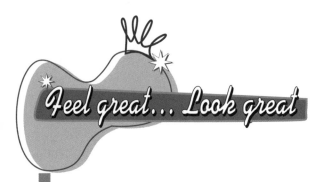

Feel great... Look great

Section Highlights

Ways to restore and repair your teeth:

◆ Fillings
◆ Crowns
◆ Root canal
◆ Fixed bridges
◆ Dental implants
◆ Partial dentures
◆ Full dentures
◆ Cosmetic dentistry
◆ Adult braces

*I*t happens so often that a dentist or physician is a great technician but not a great communicator. As patients, we are either lulled to sleep by technical, carefully placed words, or we are pressed into action by a busy physician giving life-or-death information and talking in triple speed. We feel rushed to make a decision. And afterwards we feel insecure about our choices, especially when no one has come forward with honest and easy-to-understand information. How can we make informed dental decisions when we know so little about the subject? It is easier than you think. It is all about knowing your options and finding out what is available.

In this section, we unravel the various ways the dentist can help restore your teeth and smile to the highest level of function and fit. And because you may be considering a cosmetic gift for yourself, we show dramatic age-defying and life-altering smile make-over results that can be achieved by cosmetic dentistry.

After reading this section, we think you'll find that choosing your dentistry will be easier and make a whole lot more more sense.

RESTORING YOUR NATURAL TEETH

*I*n the past five to 10 years, dentistry has jumped forward in the areas of fit, function, and appearance with space-age materials, state-of-the-art dental treatments, and computer imaging techniques. It is now more possible than ever before to restore, reshape, whiten, straighten, and sculpt new, youthful smiles while rearranging collapsing or aging facial features.

Behind every smile is a life or death function. Teeth are the first stage of digestion. Without teeth, your stomach struggles to break down and process what you eat in order to provide vitamins and nutrients to your body. And, of course, teeth play a vital role in the joy of eating certain foods. As we age, the pleasure of eating becomes paramount. Ask someone with ill-fitting dentures what bothers them the most—is it the discomfort of the dentures or not eating the foods they love? They will fervently answer the latter.

REPAIRING CAVITIES

Teeth are different than skin or bones or other parts of the body in that they do not heal on their own. Although much technical and medical progress has been made in the area of dentistry, there are simply some teeth that cannot be fixed and saved. Thankfully, in most cases, teeth can be repaired and/or restored. When dental work is necessary, a dentist strives to restore the tooth as nearly as humanly possible to its former functioning status.

Filling Teeth: What Are Your Options?

"Fillings" are a common dental procedure and easy to understand. When you get a cavity, the dentist removes the decay and fills the hole with a "filling."

Amalgam Fillings

For over 100 years, amalgams were used by dentists worldwide as the "filling of choice" for repairing teeth. An amalgam is a filling material composed of silver and mercury. But media attention has generated a growing concern (and controversy) among consumers about the health consequences of amalgam and a fear of mercury toxicity.

Sink Your Teeth into This: Research has not proved a link to any health benefits from removing amalgams from teeth. But it has been our experience that most people, when given a choice, do not want any new or additional amalgams put into their mouth.

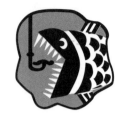

Amalgam Filling Benefits

◆ Less expensive

◆ Present fewer difficulties when getting insurance to cover the cost

Amalgam Filling Drawbacks

◆ Dark and unattractive

◆ Stain the natural tooth

◆ Expand and, over a period of years, can cause natural teeth to crack

◆ Contain mercury and silver, which can get lodged under the gum and cause blue-black discoloration on the gums

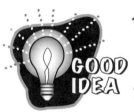

Tooth-colored Fillings

Over a decade ago, we had no proven tooth-colored dental material that could fill a hole left behind by decay and withstand the chewing forces of the teeth. Today that has changed. Tooth-colored fillings have so

---

GOOD DENTISTS WILL STAND BEHIND THEIR WORK

Completed fillings, crowns, and bridges should feel good, look good, and "clean good." Discuss any undesirable outcomes with your dentist. He or she will present you with options for making things right.

Examine the Tooth Shape and Shade

SHAPE: Does it look like a natural tooth or like a piece of Chiclets® gum? Too bulky and too white screams, *"I'm a phony!"*

SHADE: Check the shade of a tooth-colored filling (or crown, or bridge, etc.) Does it match your surrounding teeth? If not, did the doctor discuss *prior to treatment* why a color match would not be possible?

Do a Tongue Test on Dental Work

Does it feel good?

✔ Smooth to the tongue

✔ Comfortable to your bite

Is it going to clean easily?

✔ Won't trap food

✔ Won't get hungup on your floss

✔ Sensitive to brush

much improved because of superior high-tech dental materials and dental techniques that many dentists no longer offer amalgam fillings. Our "filling of choice" is now the tooth-colored restoration.

Tooth-colored Filling Benefits

◆ Look like a tooth

◆ Help to strengthen the tooth

◆ Do not stain teeth or gums

◆ Seals the tooth

◆ Does not expand or cause the tooth to fracture

Tooth-colored Filling Drawbacks

◆ Take more time for both patient and doctor

◆ Are more expensive

Often insurance will not pay for the cost difference between an amalgam filling and a tooth-colored filling.

Inlays and Onlays

Inlays and onlays aren't considered fillings because they are made in a dental laboratory. They aren't crowns either because they fit on the inside of the tooth and do not cover the tooth completely. The new porcelain and plastic dental materials have, for the most part, replaced the gold inlays and onlays used by most dentists in the past.

Inlays and onlays are used at the discretion of the dentist and will depend on the dentist's training. They are stronger than other fillings and are made of a tooth-colored material which is used on the chewing surfaces of the back teeth. The new inlays and onlays work very well as an aesthetic choice. In fact, they are cosmetically superior to any other type of crown. They hold the tooth together from the inside, whereas a crown holds the tooth in place from the outside as a cover. The disadvantage is that time has not proven the strength of the new inlays and onlays compared to the proven performance of crowns.

MAKE SURE YOUR STAINLESS STEEL CROWN IS NOT A PERMANENT MOUTH GUEST!

If you are an adult with a stainless steel crown in your mouth, you need to know that the crown was meant to be worn temporarily—not to be worn forever. These crowns are pre-formed rather than custom-made and fitted for your tooth. When worn over a long period of time, they can cause dental damage.

1. Stainless steel crowns are not sealed tight around the tooth structure and can catch food underneath, irritate the gums, and cause decay and gum disease.

2. Soft material in a stainless steel temporary crown will not always withstand the biting and chewing forces of your teeth.

However, on children's primary back teeth, stainless steel is one of the treatments of choice.

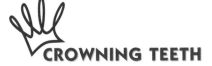
CROWNING TEETH

If part of your tooth is missing or broken off, and a "filling" cannot be supported by the remaining tooth structure, a crown will be necessary (some folks may refer to a crown as a "cap"). If your problem is a cracked tooth, the sooner it is treated and crowned, the more likely it will be saved. Once the crown is cemented on, it is stationary and works as a protective cover. The crown will add extra strength to your tooth structure and will improve the appearance of the tooth.

When Do You Need a Crown?

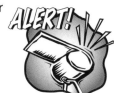

1. To strengthen a decayed, cracked or broken tooth.

2. To protect a tooth that's "at risk" for cracking. This measure helps to prevent problems such as pain and/or the need for a root canal.

3. To improve the appearance of the tooth.

4. To improve the cleansibility of a tooth or teeth.

5. After a tooth has root canal therapy.

CRACKED TEETH

Many people have teeth with natural fracture lines. These do not necessarily point to a cracked tooth. A cracked tooth usually causes pain when biting. The pain may not be constant; in fact, it often comes and goes. If you have any pain of this type or suspect a cracked tooth, be sure to call your dentist. A *strong bite* and a *weak tooth* are the perfect combination for creating a cracked or split tooth. Eventually a cracked tooth may require a root canal procedure and a crown. When a cracked tooth is suspected, the general dentist may refer the patient to an endodontist for additional diagnostic testing.

Signs and Symptoms:

✔ Often there's no constant pain but intermittent mild pain that sometimes goes away suddenly. This makes it easy to ignore or delay treatment of a cracked tooth.

✔ The tooth may be sensitive to hot or cold.

✔ When applying pressure to the tooth, it may hurt on one occasion and not the next.

What Are Your Choices?

COMBINATION PORCELAIN AND METAL CROWNS—Tooth-colored restorations typically used on the back teeth (molars).

ALL-PORCELAIN CROWN—The restoration used on teeth that show when you smile. This new technology is cosmetically superior to the old porcelain-fused-to-metal crowns because it eliminates the ugly black lines at the gum line.

GOLD CROWNS—The benchmark of function, gold crowns can be used anywhere.

Dealing with Infected Teeth

A standard comedian's punch line is to compare their worst nightmare to having a r-r-rroooot canal. Patients tell dentists the joke backwards:

"I'd rather visit my ex-husband, or go to my class reunion than get a root canal."

Root canal therapy is a much-maligned dental procedure. Once the infected tooth is treated with antibiotics, the infection subsides, and a trained specialist performs the root canal therapy, the procedure usually goes quite smoothly.

GOOD NEWS: ROOT CANAL TOOTH WITH A CROWN

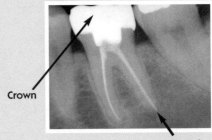

Crown

Root tip

The above image shows a good example of proper root canal therapy. The root is cleaned out down to the very tip and sealed off.

BAD NEWS: ROOT CANAL TOOTH WITHOUT A CROWN

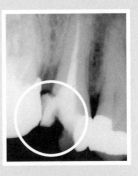

This image shows a root canal tooth that was never crowned and, as a result, the tooth broke.

What Is an Infected Tooth?

Once decay hits the nerve, a "super-infection" begins. And once the nerve is infected, bacteria creates a gas which causes pressure and throbbing, swelling pain that makes you want to run to the dentist for help. A severe toothache is one of the most painful human events possible—and an event to be avoided at all costs.

■ ■ ■ ■ ■ ■ ■ ■ ■ ■

WHAT IS AN ENDODONTIST?

An *endodontist* does root canal therapy all day long. He or she is a dentist who has received two additional years of training following graduation from dental school. Endodontists specialize in treating the soft inner tissue (the nerve) of a tooth and treating oral and facial pain.

■ ■ ■ ■ ■ ■ ■ ■ ■ ■

The Only Options when Infection Occurs:

1. Save the tooth with root canal therapy. This therapy replaces the nerve with a substance that the body will accept.

2. Lose the tooth by surgical removal. Removal results in an empty space in the gums, which can cause the bite to collapse and can place stress on the remaining teeth.

There are times when teeth cannot be restored and must be extracted. When a tooth is "too far gone" with decay, is split down the middle, or has no bone support due to gum disease, it must be removed.

Your best choice, whenever possible, is root canal therapy which will allow you to save the tooth. After treatment, it will be necessary to crown the tooth to prevent further breakage. Because the tooth no longer has blood circulation, it will become dry and brittle.

GOOD IDEA

If your dentist determines that a root canal is necessary, he or she will perform the root canal procedure. Or if the root poses a problem or you are medically compromised, the dentist will refer you to an *endodontist.*

Root canal therapy in a difficult tooth may be a difficult situation. You can ask your dentist,"Can you handle this or would it be best to refer me to an endodontist?" Our recommendation? In a difficult case, we definitely would opt for an endodontist.

REPLACING MISSING TEETH

Chapter Two

*L*et's speculate that you have just had a tooth pulled and your dentist suggests that you get a fixed bridge. Maybe you are wondering why you need to fill in the hole? Nobody can see the empty space when you smile. So what's the problem? The problem is this. When you leave an empty space in your mouth, you jeopardize the health and function of *all* your remaining teeth. It's the domino effect. And if you will remember, one way to lose teeth is when they don't fit together properly.

Teeth shift to compensate for the space left behind by the missing tooth (or teeth) and when that happens:

- ✔ Your bite gets out of harmony with your jaw joints.
- ✔ Your chewing pattern gets thrown off and puts a strain on all your remaining teeth.
- ✔ You become at risk for losing more teeth.
- ✔ Your appearance and health suffers. Tooth loss causes bone loss, and bone loss contributes to a sagging face.

A FIXED BRIDGE

A dental bridge does exactly what the word implies: it bridges across an empty space. A fixed bridge is anchored from one strong tooth to another strong tooth and fills the gap that was left by the missing tooth (or teeth).

Bridge Benefits
- ◆ A fixed bridge is stationary. You don't need to take it out at night.
- ◆ It looks like your natural teeth.
- ◆ It's comfortable and doesn't move when you're chewing.
- ◆ It anchors and supports your neighboring teeth; keeps teeth aligned; and restores your mouth to a level of prevention.

Bridge Drawbacks
There really are no drawbacks but a bridge needs to be cleaned very diligently. You will have to use a floss threader or irrigator and get under the bridge to keep plaque and bacteria from collecting.

DENTAL IMPLANTS

Many years of dental research, combined with the pioneering efforts of some truly dedicated dentists and the medical strides in joint replacement surgery, have made a contribution to the successful leap forward for dental implants. Today, titanium implant systems are well tolerated in the mouth and are a viable option for many people who are missing one or all of their teeth.

What Are Dental Implants?

Dental implants are the nearest thing to natural tooth function available in dentistry at this time. Using the same principles and material used in joint replacement surgery, dental implants are securely anchored into bone and will attach to single or multiple replacement teeth. Implants are also used to anchor full-mouth dentures.

Benefits of Implants

◆ Implants feel more comfortable, secure, and natural than removable tooth replacements such as a partial denture.

◆ Implants allow you to eat what you want.

◆ Implants give you the confidence to freely laugh and smile with ease.

◆ Implants will stop the jawbone from shrinking, which in turn stops premature facial aging.

Things to Consider about Dental Implants

The decision to get a dental implant requires a firm commitment and a strong desire for good fit and confident function,

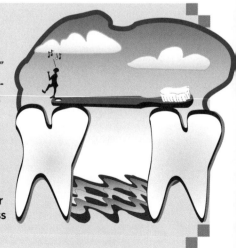

A BRIDGE OVER TROUBLED WATERS

Here's a typical dental office scenario:

The dentist says, *"You need a fixed bridge here."*

And your answer is, *"These teeth have been missing for years. Why get a bridge now?"* What most people don't realize is that dental damage has been progressing slowly over a period of time. When teeth are missing on one side of your mouth, the teeth on the opposite side are getting overworked. The extra stress puts the teeth at risk. If you don't put in a fixed bridge or dental implant before permanent damage weakens or destroys the remaining teeth, you end up with less comfortable options.

IMPLANTS: HOLDING YOUR SMILE TOGETHER

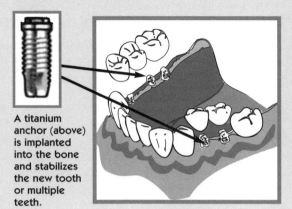

A titanium anchor (above) is implanted into the bone and stabilizes the new tooth or multiple teeth.

Versatility, function, and appearance are important assets for people who have lost teeth. An implant can hold a single tooth, multiple teeth, or even a full-mouth denture. The illustration shows the two-step process of dental implants. First, a titanium anchor is set into the bone. Later, the necessary bridge, denture or tooth is attached to the implant.

as well as an attractive smile. Getting dental implants can mean several hours in the dentist's chair extended over many months. The work is complex and costly. Not every dentist is capable of installing dental implants. In fact, it is one of the most complex procedures in dentistry. Implant dentistry is not yet a specialty, so when considering this option, it is vitally important to find a dentist with extensive dental implant experience.

Depending on the case, multiple implants can reach a substantial cost—as much as the price of a high-end vehicle. Insurance benefits will usually cover only a small portion of the cost.

Who Is a Good Dental Implant Candidate?

Lifestyle habits can work for or against your implant success. According to the Academy of General Dentistry (AGD), implants have a current success rate of 70 to 90 percent after 10 years. Just as with any surgery, good health and a strong immune system are always positive starting points.

But a good dentist will interview you extensively and discuss both your medical background and your lifestyle habits.

- ◆ Healthy gums are important for the surgical healing process.
- ◆ Adequate bone support will be necessary.
- ◆ Smoking will compromise the success of the implant.

Where Do Implants Work the Best?

For those who have already lost teeth, dental implants are becoming a popular alternative to bridges or partial dentures because they can:

- ◆ Support a single-tooth replacement.
- ◆ Support multiple-tooth replacements. It is possible to replace all teeth with dental implants in place of getting full-mouth dentures.
- ◆ Support removable dentures. This is very helpful on a lower denture which tends to get knocked out by the tongue and the movement of the lower jaw.

PARTIAL DENTURES

What Is a Partial Denture?

A partial denture is a removable dental appliance that replaces missing teeth. In other words, unlike the fixed bridge and the dental implant, you will need to put it into your mouth and take it out to clean. The artificial teeth are held in place in your mouth with support from your teeth, jawbone, and gums.

Deciding to Get a Partial Denture

A partial denture is necessary for the same reason that you need a bridge—you have a missing tooth or teeth. We don't, however, recommend it as an easy and cheap option for replacing a salvageable tooth.

You must consider your options before making a decision. Is budget a big concern? Or is comfort a must-have? Think hard about what you can tolerate. For some, adjusting to a removable dental appliance is not possible. In order to make the right decision for you, carefully read through the following reality checks.

Choose a partial denture when:

- ✔ A fixed bridge is not an option because you are missing the necessary strong anchoring teeth.
- ✔ A dental implant is not an option for anchoring teeth.
- ✔ You need to replace too many teeth and/or budget is a concern.

AGE-DEFYING ADVICE

As the rest of your body ages, so do your teeth. Can we put on the brakes and slow down the aging process in your mouth and face? You bet! Plastic surgery isn't the only option for a sagging face. Keeping your smile white and bright and your mouth and teeth healthy and functioning will add years to your life while subtracting years from your face. An ounce of dental prevention is worth a pound of plastic surgery.

Three things that make you look older faster:

1. Gum disease

2. Missing, worn down, broken, yellow, or stained teeth

3. Ill-fitting dentures or bridges

Will a Partial Denture Work for You?

✔ Do you require comfort? Hooks, wires, metal, plastic, and food getting stuck—does that sound comfortable to you?

✔ How adaptable are you? An upper partial can be a problem for people who gag easily. The lower partial takes some getting used to because your lower jaw and tongue move constantly in reaction to the "foreign object."

✔ Some people never do adjust and the partial sits in a drawer.

✔ If you sing or play a reed or brass instrument or if your job requires public speaking, you may have difficulty adjusting.

The Budget Benefits

You may need to make a decision based on economics. The reality is that the only reason to choose a partial denture over a dental implant, if that's an option for you, is when finances are a major issue and/or your ability to adapt to the removable appliance is good.

◆ You get multiple teeth replaced for one price.

◆ A partial has remodeling possibilities—in some instances you can add more teeth to the partial at a later date.

The Drawbacks

◆ Annoying—Food gets caught under the denture.

◆ Uncomfortable—If not fitted properly, the denture will move around.

◆ Embarrassing—People don't like the thought of a removable tooth, and metal clasps on partials may be visible.

◆ An adjustment period—It takes several dental visits to adjust the fit.

◆ A nuisance—Easy to lose.

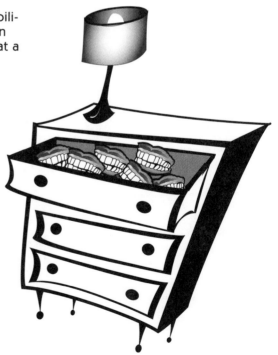

FULL-MOUTH DENTURES

We believe and strongly suggest you keep and cherish every tooth in your mouth that can be saved.

Everything about a denture is a drawback unless you just don't have a choice. Studies show that you lose over 75% of your chewing pressure when you lose all your natural teeth and must depend on dentures.

- ◆ Chewing pressure with natural teeth ranges from 55 pounds per square inch to 280 pounds per square inch.

- ◆ Chewing pressure with full-mouth dentures ranges from 22 to 47 pounds per square inch.

That's quite a significant reduction. Your frail, 90-year-old aunt who has all her teeth has a more powerful bite than a strong 200-pound man with dentures. Once your teeth are gone, the nerves and ligaments in your mouth no longer report to the brain to tell how hard to chew. And to add insult to injury, the jaw muscles become weak because they are no longer getting their daily workout. Over time, the cheeks sink in as the muscles get weaker. This is why the face ages prematurely in people who wear full-mouth dentures.

AUDREY'S NEW DENTURES MIRROR HER SMILE FROM 25 YEARS AGO

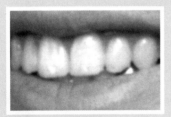

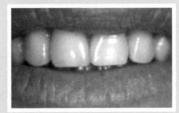

Audrey's new denture—Restored her youthful smile, but it will never replace her beautiful natural teeth.

Audrey's high school yearbook smile.

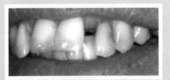

Audrey 25 years later, before dentures.

Audrey's story:
"I wish I would have known..."

Twenty-five years after high school, Audrey's smile was destroyed. It never occurred to her that the "new space" developing over time between her teeth was due to advanced gum and bone disease. Audrey believed that "feeling no dental pain" was a sign that her teeth were okay, so she saw no reason to go to the dentist. By the time she sought help, it was too late to save her teeth. Audrey was devastated by the news.

What Is a Full-mouth Denture?

A set of full-mouth dentures can basically be described as two pieces of plastic that have a really big job to perform. After all, they literally become the infrastructure of your mouth.

Those who must wear removable dentures face daily anxiety about performing even the most ordinary of tasks. Many denture wearers feel they must be continually vigilant about the security of their "teeth," which probably explains why billions of fear-driven dollars are spent each year on denture adhesives.

Some people on the other hand have no problems with their dentures. The "Catch 22" is that you won't know which camp you are in until you actually lose all your teeth. *When that happens, there is no going back.*

Why Full-Mouth Dentures?

If you and your dentist determine that you need dentures, your dentist should complete a comprehensive examination. Be sure to do this *before you act on that decision* because there's no turning

WHAT A DENTURE LOVER IS REALLY SAYING

Why do some patients say, "Getting my teeth taken out was the best thing I ever did?" Because they were in a lot of pain from infection. Their teeth and gums hurt all the time. The prospect of dentures was a healthier choice than keeping their teeth. So the fact is, they had no choice. Once the infected teeth were gone, the patients became infection-free. The healing process began and they felt better from head to toe. This is certainly no endorsement for getting dentures. It only shows how patients can make lemonade out of lemons. And we applaud them for adjusting to their dentures.

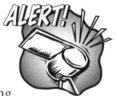

WHEN YOUR DENTIST SAYS NO TO DENTURES

People tell us, *"I'm tired of spending money on my teeth"* or *"I don't want to worry about my teeth. Pull them all out."* They believe if they have no teeth, they will have no more problems and will escape going to the dentist. The trouble is when you trade in an old set of problems for a set of dentures, new challenges are just beginning. You don't avoid going to the dentist; in fact, you go often for different reasons.

Can your teeth be saved? When the answer is yes, but your budget says no, ask yourself, "Is pulling a tooth really cheaper than spending more than a thousand dollars for a root canal and crown?" Weigh your decision carefully. Even if the math seems obvious, you don't know all the consequences and repercussions of losing teeth. No amount of money can ever get your teeth back. Before you decide that the dentist is just trying to make money off you, *give your teeth a fighting chance.* Give your dentist an opportunity to thoroughly evaluate your dental situation.

back later. Remember, seeing is believing. Ask the dentist to show you the x-rays or images that tell the story of your teeth and explain to you *in a way that you can understand* why you need dentures. Have your dentist point out the amount of bone loss and decay that has destroyed your teeth. If you do not fully understand your x-rays or the dentist has not explained them to your satisfaction and you have not had a comprehensive dental exam, get a second opinion.

When Dentures Are a Must, Make the Best of the Experience

Adapting to dentures will challenge your "learning curve." No set of dentures can replace or feel as right as your God-given teeth (even if they were not in great dental condition). Change is hard, but a good attitude will go a long way to getting you adjusted to dentures. The irony is that it is more important than ever now—when you have no teeth left—to have a trusting relationship with your dentist.

Discuss with Your Dentist:

◆ What is it that you liked or disliked about other people's dentures?

◆ What is it you liked or disliked about your former dentures?

The number one criteria for a good denture will be that it looks good to you. Teeth must be placed in the right position to make you look natural whether you are smiling a small relaxed smile or grinning from ear to ear.

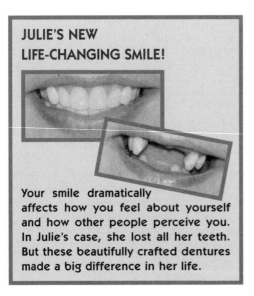

JULIE'S NEW LIFE-CHANGING SMILE!

Your smile dramatically affects how you feel about yourself and how other people perceive you. In Julie's case, she lost all her teeth. But these beautifully crafted dentures made a big difference in her life.

Getting a Good Fit on Dentures

The dentist is responsible for fitting the dentures correctly. People who wear dentures mistakenly believe (thanks to all the commercials) that they must also wear dental adhesives. In most cases, this is not true. If your dentures fit properly, dental adhesive should not be necessary (unless you do not have enough supporting bone in your mouth).

The best use of dental adhesives is for short-term use during the stage when you are wearing "immediate (interim) dentures." This may be necessary while waiting for your full-mouth dentures to be made. Keep in mind that dental adhesives can create a new set of problems with prolonged use.

A denture does not fit well when it:

✔ Hurts

✔ Makes a clicking sound

✔ Causes lisping or whistling sounds

✔ Doesn't help fill out your cheeks

✔ Doesn't look good

✔ Looks like "false teeth"

✔ Is loose and falls out

✔ Causes sores on your gums

Wearing full-mouth dentures does not mean that you are "out of the woods" when it comes to seeing a dental professional. You will still need:

◆ Oral cancer screening

◆ Dental examination for any infection on the gums

TRUE CONFESSIONS

One hot summer night, Mac Lee was dining out at a Texas-style Bar-B-Q restaurant with a friend who has full-mouth dentures. Observing that the cowboy seemed to be having no problem chewing the ribs and corn on the cob, Lee brought up the subject of dentures. The cowboy was one of the more fortunate folks who could eat almost anything due to the dental implants securing his lower denture.

Finally Mac asked a very personal question. What amount of money would this cowboy pay to get his natural teeth back if they were in perfect working condition? The leather-skinned rancher thought about it for half a second. "$50,000," he hollered. No chump change for a good ole' boy living on a fixed income.

Chapter Three

COSMETIC DENTISTRY
Bright, White, Straight, Glitzy, and "In Your Face" Smiles!

*O*ur psyche is greatly damaged by a smile with missing teeth and unbecoming dental mishaps. Self-confidence, speech, movement, and spontaneity are essential parts of our *chi*, our inner self, our beliefs, and our understanding of who we are. The fact is if you have all the information you need, as well as the money and the desire to cosmetically improve your smile, the dental materials, artistry, and technical talent are certainly available.

Yet thousands of dollars and scads of time is spent on weight-lifting, moisturizing, toning, and surgically altering facial structure while the appearance and health of teeth are overlooked or given a token whitening.

Few things are more uncomfortable than watching a person self-consciously conceal a smile behind his or her hand. Positioning his or her lips to hide the secret, broken condition of his/her teeth, the person's body language announces, "That's enough, no more, don't make me laugh." It's as if being too happy is too painful.

"IT ALL STARTED WITH A BROKEN TOOTH!"

No one hid her smile more often than Joleen Jackson, one of our authors. Today, she openly smiles and laughs confidently (especially at her own jokes!). Those who knew her before will tell you what a difference Joleen's smile makeover has made. But it wasn't easy and it didn't all happen overnight. It took a personal commitment with an investment of money (comparable to the cost of a mid-size car), time, and a combination of orthodontal and cosmetic dentistry to get the job done.

It all started with a broken tooth. Joleen went to the dentist and learned that she needed a root canal and a crown. Raising three daughters, she was on a limited income, had a busy schedule and wasn't really aware of (or even interested in) her dental options. Eight years later, she went to work in a dental office with Dr. Mac Lee and finally learned her dental options.

FIND OUT ALL YOUR OPTIONS

You don't have to work at a dental office to find out all your dental options. Our main purpose for writing this book is to arm consumers with the information they need to make wise and informed dental decisions. The more you know, the better your chances of finding the right person to become the caretaker of your mouth.

Joleen didn't immediately have the money to pay for her restorative dentistry. But once she found out what was available to her, she decided what she wanted to do and devised a plan. Over time, she saved the necessary amount of money, and nine years ago Dr. Lee completed her cosmetic restoration.

When family and friends learned what she was going to do, they commented that her teeth didn't look that bad. But they didn't see what Joleen saw while working in the dental office—patients whose lives had been totally transformed by cosmetic changes to their smiles.

After her smile was completely restored Joleen said,

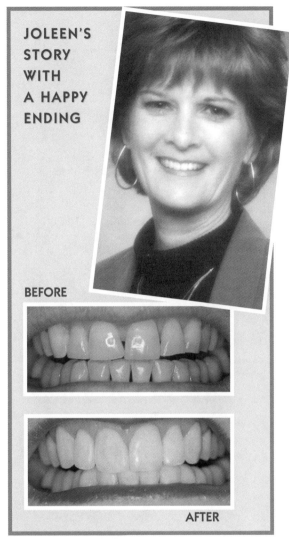

JOLEEN'S STORY WITH A HAPPY ENDING

BEFORE

AFTER

"My only regret was that I didn't do it sooner! It's cheaper to hide your smile than to fix it, but it feels great to look richer, younger, and more attractive. Maybe it isn't fair that we live in a society that judges people by their looks, but after my teeth were restored I discovered that they do. People see me today as a more competent professional."

Joleen "Before"

A comprehensive dental exam revealed the following problems for Joleen. She complained that every time she went to the dentist it seemed that she always needed more dental work done that cost a lot of money. But she didn't completely understand (or hear) why the work was necessary.

JOLEEN'S SMILE BEFORE

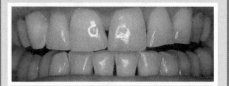

Joleen's teeth didn't fit together properly. If you look at the "before" picture, you can see that her teeth were slanted and not straight up and down. They were also shorter on one side than on the other.

JOLEEN'S SMILE AFTER

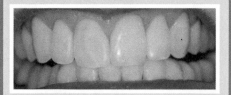

Dr. Lee restored her teeth with all-porcelain crowns. In addition to looking great, they make it easy for Joleen to floss and keep clean.

Typical of an early baby boomer, Joleen's first visit to the dentist was at age seven, when her lower six-year molars had to be removed due to massive decay. Her diet as a child included a high amount of sugar. She also had other dental problems:

- ◆ Her tooth-grinding was causing the teeth to wear down.

- ◆ Her teeth were yellow and stained.

- ◆ Her remaining molars were cracked from large, expanding amalgam fillings.

- ◆ In the back of her front teeth, she had large, difficult-to-keep-clean, "old" white fillings.

- ◆ Joleen's gum recession made her look "long in the tooth"— older than her real age.

Joleen "After"

Joleen describes it best,

"I spent time and money to get the results that I personally wanted and needed for my mouth. I don't like things left up in the air or untended. This was a dream come true for me. Because of the restoration, my teeth are so easy to keep clean and, barring an accident, I never have to worry about needing any major dental work again, if I keep up my daily home care. No more nagging little voice in my head saying, 'You better get to the dentist.' I do, however, get my teeth cleaned every three months to protect my investment. Also, to protect my porcelain crowns from my tooth-grinding, I wear a plastic night guard to bed."

Be Aware of "Quick Fix" Makeovers

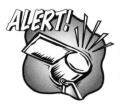

Because quality restorations take time, expensive lab work, and the proper equipment, cosmetic dentistry is a very exacting job. Treatment involves time, commitment, and money. So if a dentist's estimate of time and cost sounds too good to be true, it probably is too good to be true.

How Does Your Smile Measure Up?

First impressions leave powerful, lingering images. People with beautiful, becoming smiles make memorable entrances. They are covered with compliments, promoted, and even over-paid. In today's "supermodel" environment, drop-dead smiles are a valuable asset, while teeth that don't look so good can work as a liability and an unwarranted strike against you in a sometimes critical world. A crooked or gummy smile with missing, crowded teeth will override other attractive facial features. But you don't have to be born with a great smile. You can buy it.

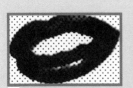

RATE YOUR SMILE

On a scale of one to ten—one being not so good and ten being great—*circle* the number that describes *your* smile.

✔ **"I don't smile a lot because of my teeth."**
  1 2 3 4 5 6 7 8 9 10

✔ **"I hide my smile and cover my teeth when I laugh."**
  1 2 3 4 5 6 7 8 9 10

✔ **"I wish my teeth were whiter."**
  1 2 3 4 5 6 7 8 9 10

✔ **"I wish my teeth weren't so crooked."**
  1 2 3 4 5 6 7 8 9 10

✔ **"I guess my teeth are okay."**
  1 2 3 4 5 6 7 8 9 10

✔ **"I wear a moustache to hide my teeth."**
  1 2 3 4 5 6 7 8 9 10

✔ **"I don't know. I never look in the mirror."**
  1 2 3 4 5 6 7 8 9 10

✔ **"I have a knock-em-dead gorgeous smile!"**
  AUTOMATIC 10 POINTS!

BEAUTIFUL SMILES SOLD HERE!

Look what can be achieved with cosmetic dentistry.

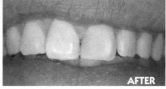

CRACKED OR BROKEN TEETH

A traumatic blow to the mouth changed a beautiful smile into a "nightmare."

New dental restorative material and advanced technology allow dentists to bond tooth-colored plastics directly to a chipped tooth to restore a damaged smile.

GAPS BETWEEN TEETH

During tooth development not all teeth are correctly formed. Notice that in the "before" photo, spaces between the teeth resemble pegs. The teeth are smaller at the biting than at the gumline.

Cosmetic dentistry, using all porcelain crowns and laminates, created a whiter, younger, and healthier smile.

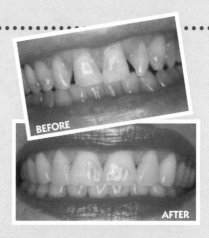

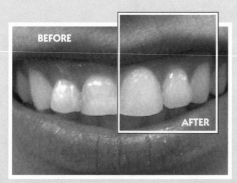

GUMMY SMILE

For unknown reasons, teeth do not always fully erupt out of the gums. The outcome is a gummy smile. The treatment is a simple procedure of removing the extra gum and exposing the right amount of tooth.

The inset at the left shows that more tooth and less exposed gum create a prettier smile.

PROFESSIONAL WHITENING OPTIONS

✔ **Same-Day Whitening**

Safe, Quick, and Easy Bleaching. This type of professional bleaching done in the dental office gives you "immediate gratification."

✔ **Two-Week Bleaching**

Safe, but Time-Consuming Home Kit. Your dentist will take an impression of your teeth and customize a mouthpiece to go along with your professional whitening kit. Use the kit at home for about two weeks and then occasionally after that to boost your whitening job.

It's important to get your teeth bleached prior to any cosmetic restoration work, or you will risk a different color match, if you get your teeth bleached at a later time.

(The American Dental Association has not approved any over-the-counter bleaching products. Talk to your dentist or hygienist before using any of these products.)

Looking for a Good Cosmetic Dentist

When you are searching for a cosmetic dentist, research becomes critically important for many reasons. Cosmetic dentistry is not a recognized specialty at this point. Therefore, any dentist can perform cosmetic dentistry and a gazillion doctors are advertising "smile makeovers."

When it comes to plastic surgery, most people would do major research before choosing a plastic surgeon to reshape their face. The same advice should hold true when getting your smile restored. You don't want just any dentist to alter and reshape your teeth. In other words, let your "fingers do the walking" through the phone book, but don't stop there. Plan on doing your homework. The first step is to ask for a referral from trusted acquaintances whose new smiles you admire.

When interviewing dentists, beware of the "cosmetic" dentist who is only concerned about the way your teeth look. Aesthetics cannot come at the expense of having a healthy mouth and a harmonious bite. A good architect will tell you that it

BLEACHING: WHEN ONLY WHITE IS RIGHT FOR YOUR TEETH

Bleaching your teeth is a simple way to update a smile. Over time, teeth become discolored from age or continuous exposure to tea, coffee, red wine, dark colas, and tobacco. These stains go deep, permeating the surface of the tooth's enamel. In order to get teeth really white and remove the stains, it is necessary to penetrate below the surface of the enamel. If you want your teeth whiter, ask your dentist about bleaching.

is unwise to build mansions on cesspools, and a good restorative dentist understands the fallacy of doing expensive cosmetic improvements on teeth that are missing a healthy foundation due to gum disease or decay, or on teeth that do not fit together properly.

The dentist who will help you the most is the one who is already a good dentist and routinely does a comprehensive examination. In addition, the dentist:

♦ Should have attended advanced studies in occlusion (how the teeth fit together).

♦ Should be skilled in the use of the new cosmetic technology and should use this skill along with repairing and restoring teeth to fit, function, and comfort.

Ask the Right Questions

Be sure to communicate your goals and expectations to the dentist. You won't upset her (or him) and she will get a better understanding of how to accomplish what you want. Some questions to ask are:

♦ What advanced education courses in occlusion (bite relationship) have you taken? What advanced courses have you attended for cosmetic dentistry (some professionals use the term "esthetics")?

♦ How well will the cosmetic work that you are recommending for my smile fit in with my existing bite?

♦ How closely do you work with your dental laboratory? Do you and your lab have the same type of training? Will you be using photographs of my mouth to communicate my special needs to the lab?

♦ Does your lab use all of the latest technology and do their technicians work under a microscope?

♦ Do you have any "before" and "after" photographs of your work?

♦ Do you have a list of satisfied cosmetic patients I could contact?

Most importantly, trust your instincts.

ARE YOU A CANDIDATE FOR ADULT BRACES?

It is estimated that one out of every five wearers of braces is over the age of 18. Yet, many adults are unaware that they are still candidates for braces. The process involved in tooth movement is the same in both adults and children. However, because an adult's facial bones are no longer growing, certain corrections cannot be accomplished with braces alone. Dentists achieve dramatic facial changes with the combined approach of surgery and orthodontics. Get an orthodontic evaluation. The health of your teeth, gums, and supporting bone will be the most important factor in determining your prospects for improving your smile and your dental health with braces.

SPACE-AGE COMFORT

Space-age technology has streamlined braces, making them more comfortable and less noticeable. They also require less time in the doctor's office. There are, however, a few inconveniences. Certain sticky, brittle treats are off limits. And your mouth may be a little tender after adjustments. But you'll adjust quickly—after all you are a grown-up.

The Benefits of Braces

Braces can do more than just give you a great smile that helps you snag a raise at work and a date with that girl you see at the coffee shop every morning. When you treat orthodontic problems, you also improve the health of your teeth and gums. Take a look at some of the dental problems braces can help to address:

- ◆ Crowded teeth are hard to clean and maintain and, in time, can contribute to decay, gum disease, and eventual tooth loss.

- ◆ When teeth don't fit together properly, the result can be abnormal wear on tooth surfaces, difficulty in chewing, damage to supporting bone and gum tissue, and tooth loss.

- ◆ Jaw joint (TMJ) pain and associated headaches sometimes can be attributed to crooked teeth and incorrect bites.

- ◆ When spaces due to missing teeth are present, teeth can be moved to accommodate future fixed bridges or dental implants.

Selecting Your Orthodontist

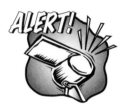

When you are looking for an orthodontist, you want to make sure that he or she will do a "diagnostic records exam." As you are making your calls, inquire whether this exam is a standard practice in that dental office.

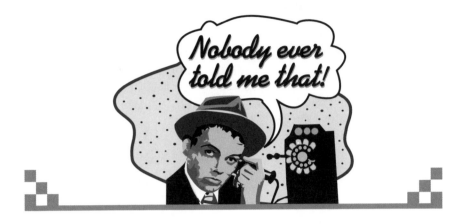

Nobody ever told me that!

- You will look older faster with the following dental problems: gum disease; missing, stained or broken teeth; and ill-fitting dentures or bridges.

- Amalgam fillings can expand and, over a period of years, cause natural teeth to crack.

- Tooth-colored fillings look natural and do not expand or cause the tooth to fracture.

- A crown is recommended for several reasons. One reason is to re-establish the biting surfaces of the teeth. Another may be to prevent an "at risk" tooth from cracking.

- Teeth that have root canal therapy should be crowned because the tooth will dry up and possibly break.

- Root canal therapy is always your best and healthiest option, rather than pulling the tooth.

- When root canal therapy is necessary on a difficult tooth ask your dentist, *"If it were your tooth, Doc, would you have an endodontist perform your root canal therapy?"*

- When a missing tooth leaves a space in your mouth, your chewing pattern gets thrown off and puts a strain on all your remaining teeth. As a result, you are at risk for losing more teeth.

- You can secure a single tooth, multiple teeth, and even full-mouth removable dentures with dental implants.

- Some people never adjust to a partial denture and it ends up sitting in a drawer. An upper partial can be a problem for people who gag.

- From a budget standpoint, a partial denture may be a good option. It also has "remodeling" possibilities, if you need more teeth added to it in the future.

- A 200-pound man with full-mouth dentures has less chewing force than his 90-year-old aunt who has all her teeth.

- Dental adhesives are meant to be used short-term, not as a substitute for ill-fitting dentures. If your dentures don't fit properly, call your dentist. You may need to get your dentures "re-lined."

- Over time, teeth can become discolored from age or continuous exposure to tea, coffee, red wine, dark colas, and tobacco. These stains go deep into the surface of the tooth. In order to get teeth really white, talk to your dentist about a professional whitening that will penetrate the tooth's enamel.

- Sometimes teeth do not fully "erupt" out of the gum and the outcome is a "gummy smile." In many cases, this can be fixed by a simple cosmetic surgical procedure.

- New dental restorative material and advanced technology allow dentists to bond tooth-colored plastics directly to a chipped tooth to restore a damaged smile.

- Many adults are unaware that they are still candidates for braces. When you treat orthodontic problems, you also improve the health of your teeth and gums. Orthodontia is not for appearance only.

SECTION VI:

MOUTH CARE FITNESS
Preventing Dental Problems

Beauty school taught me everything except how to take care of my teeth!

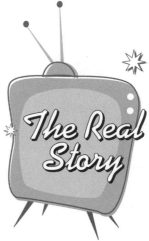

Rumor

Getting old means going bald, getting a potbelly and wearing "false teeth." That is what happened to my dad and grandpa. So, I figure I'll be another "chip off the old block."

A family history of dental neglect doesn't need to follow you into the millennium. You can avoid false teeth if you practice good dental prevention. The potbelly and going bald? Well, that's another story.

The Real Story

Keeping your mouth in shape

Section Highlights

◆ Judge your hygiene cleaning quality

◆ High-tech hygiene

◆ Authors' dental portraits

◆ Cleaning targets for gums and teeth

◆ Floss is your friend

◆ Mouth care to fit your dental profile

*Y*our smile is an integral part of your personal identity. It's your central tool of self-expression. It is the focus of how you appear to others, reflecting the structure of your face, the way you speak, and how you express emotion. A smile reveals happiness and confidence and frames one of your most precious possessions—your teeth. A smile is the final accessory that completes every outfit you wear. It is your personal signature. It signals how much you care for your mouth, teeth, gums, and yourself.

Do you collect something precious? Have you found a cherished treasure, searched for fossils, or studied fine wine? Then you understand that the stronger your passion and level of interest, the wiser you become and the more energy you spend pursuing the next coveted treasure for your collection.

Your teeth are also a prized possession. The more you understand about how to care for your mouth—what tools work best and the reasons you use them—the better you'll care for it. In this last section, we strive to motivate you to achieve your personal best. Our aim is to coach you to the highest prevention level possible for your dental health. To demonstrate our team spirit, we share our own three distinct mouth fitness stories. Using our panoramic x-rays to illustrate our individual dental histories, each of us will give you the highlights of our teeth-cleaning challenges and our daily routines.

In the dental health Olympics, your mouth must be in tip-top shape, and for this event you are the most valuable player. Your dentist and your hygienist are also key team members, handing you the baton and coaching you across the finish line where you reap the rewards.

YOUR HYGIENIST
A Dental Prevention Specialist

*W*e know that an unhealthy mouth slows you down, makes you feel tired, saps your body's defenses, and lowers your resistance to disease. A mouthful of neglect can create a long and bumpy road, and the return trip back to healthy teeth and gums can devour your precious time and earnings. It is a road you don't need to travel, if you follow proper preventive measures. Savvy dental consumers strive to stay healthy and make prevention a priority.

Dental prevention is the healthiest, most cost-effective way to care for your teeth and gums—and it takes so little time. The ultimate, daily mouth care routine may take only 15 minutes a day and will consist of brushing and flossing after every meal and before bedtime. That's five workouts a day at only three minutes each. If it's that easy, why do we resist doing what needs to be done? Well, change takes effort, and any lifestyle alteration must be done again and again until it becomes a habit and a part of a daily routine.

THE HYGIENIST AND PREVENTIVE SERVICES

Let's assume that you have found Dr. Right, received a comprehensive dental exam, and had a lifelong treatment plan established. If it is necessary to repair broken teeth, fillings, decay or any disease that irritates the gums, the dentist will complete these repairs and restore the teeth to a good condition, ready for prevention. What follows next is a plan for on-going dental health, realistic disease and decay prevention, and mouth care goals.

Hygienists are prevention specialists who are licensed and trained in prevention and

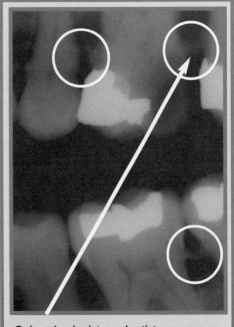

Only a hygienist or dentist can remove this calcified plaque. This calculus looks like barnacles.

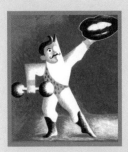

GET A WEB SITE CLEANING BOOST

The American Dental Hygiene Assoc. (ADHA) and the American Dental Assoc. (ADA) have Web sites that provide useful consumer information. The commercial product sites highlight mouth care tools and aids. A few sites also give brushing and flossing demonstrations.

www.adha.org
www.ada.org.
www.ihatedentists.com
www.ora5.com
www.oralb.com
www.colgate.com
www.glidefloss.com
www.crestsmiles.com

intervention. When infection is present in the gums and bone, they remove the offending bacteria, calculus and tartar on the teeth, above and below the gum line. If plaque hangs around long enough to calcify, only a dental professional can remove the hard deposits. This removal requires a trained hygienist with special tools to get the job done right. (See the image shown on page 149.) Once the teeth and gums are infection-free, the hygienist works to prevent any further gum infection and tooth decay. In other words, the hygienist is responsible for a whole lot more than just "polishing teeth." (Of course, they do that, too!)

Screening for signs of illness is also a part of the hygienist's preventive services. Signs and symptoms of potentially life-threatening disease can appear first in the mouth and can be detected at an early stage. Some signs and symptoms include oral lesions and lumps in the throat and neck, as well as evidence of bulimia and diabetes, to list just a few. The hygienist is in a position to detect disease risk factors and signs and symptoms while taking your medical history and doing your oral screening. Although hygienists do not diagnose disease, they do report their observations to the dentist and, when necessary, urge patients to see their physician.

Meet Your Personal Smile Coach

The fastest way to achieve any exercise and fitness goal is with a personal trainer. The same rules apply with your mouth care. Your dental hygienist is also your personal hygiene trainer and smile coach. When you have a problem mastering a brushing or flossing technique, your hygienist will walk you through the problem. A dedicated hygiene coach doesn't lecture. She or he listens to your concerns and discusses your lifestyle habits without judging. As your personal prevention trainer, your coach should motivate, educate, and help you stay the course. The hygienist should get you involved with your at-home brushing and flossing success.

Get Involved with Your Hygiene Progress

When you understand the value of keeping your mouth clean and your gums in good shape, the more motivated and committed you become in caring for your teeth and gums. It is important to take responsibility for developing good hygiene habits. The pay-off is that important. Healthy teeth will chew more comfortably, which, in turn, helps promote good nutrition. And healthy gums will hold your teeth in place and prevent dental infection from entering the bloodstream and threatening vital organs in your body.

Let Your Hygienist Know

Say that you want to be involved in your mouth care progress. Show your interest and ask your hygienist:

✔ Are there any areas in my mouth that I am missing during my brushing routine?

✔ Am I flossing correctly? Will you show me how to floss more effectively in areas that I am missing?

✔ Do I need to use fluoride gel on my teeth (due to sensitive teeth or decay)?

✔ Is it necessary for me to brush with toothpaste?

✔ What brand of toothpaste do you recommend?

✔ Do I need to use an electric toothbrush? If so, what do you recommend?

✔ Do I need to use an oral irrigation device at home (a good idea if you have gingivitis or gum disease)?

✔ How often should I get my teeth cleaned (every 3, 4, 6, or 12 months)?

✔ Is a regular cleaning sufficient or do I need a deep scaling to remove the calculus from below the gum line?

✔ Do I need to clean my tongue? Is plaque and food trapped on my tongue? Can you show me how to clean it off?

Whenever I Get My Teeth Cleaned, It Hurts!

Some people avoid getting their teeth professionally cleaned because it hurts. Or they complain that a week or two after a hygiene appointment their mouths will continue to hurt. What is going on? When teeth are sensitive or gums are infected or if you haven't had a professional cleaning in a long time, a professional cleaning can be uncomfortable.

GOOD IDEA

But you have nothing to fear. Two pain-relieving solutions are available. A special numbing mouth rinse can be administered before the teeth cleaning begins. Or some patients receive nitrous oxide during the cleaning procedure. Don't, however, measure the quality of a professional cleaning by how much it may or may not hurt. Pain is no indication that you are getting a better, more thorough job.

How Do You Judge the Quality of a Professional Cleaning?

Today, your dental hygienist can offer modern technology and comforts that make the process of teeth cleaning more efficient. A good, professional hygienist will concentrate on cleaning the two target areas—the gums and the teeth. Although there is really no "gold standard" that a consumer can use to measure the quality of a professional cleaning, there are a few gauges you can go by. During your professional cleaning, you can expect your hygienist to:

◆ Perform an oral cancer screening. This includes looking inside the mouth for any lesions and checking for any abnormalities around the throat and neck area.

HIGH-TECH HYGIENE

Hygienists have modern technology at their fingertips, which makes professional cleanings more efficient and patient-friendly. Here's a list of high-tech hygiene tools and materials. (Not all dental practices will have all of this equipment, but the list below forecasts the future of technology in the area of hygiene.)

☑ MAGNIFICATION EYEWEAR—Allows the hygienist to detect tiny problem areas on the teeth and gums. Do all hygienists wear these? No. Should they? We think so.

☑ NUMBING MOUTH RINSE—Before a professional teeth cleaning, the patient uses the mouth rinse to help diminish pain and/or discomfort caused by sensitive teeth or gums.

☑ ULTRA-SONIC SCALER—Uses ultrasonic sound waves and vibrations to remove calculus.

☑ FLUORIDE—Trays, gels, tablets, and rinses help prevent decay, and tooth sensitivity. Fluoride is available only in dental offices.

☑ NEW MEDICINES AND DELIVERY SYSTEMS—Advances in medicine allow medication to get directly into the infected area when treating gum and bone disease.

- Take and process x-rays.

- Discuss a variety of home-care tools that can give you the desired cleaning results you want for your mouth. The products may be available in the dental office or at your local stores.

- Give you hygiene instructions that are tailored to fit the condition and needs of your teeth and gums.

And after a good, thorough cleaning the hygienist should:

- Floss your teeth before polishing them to make sure the root surfaces are smooth and the calculus and tartar are completely removed.

- Check the root surfaces with a thin instrument to make sure that the area between the teeth and below the gum line is smooth and there are no clicking sounds of leftover calculus.

WHO CLEANS YOUR TEETH?

Who should give your teeth a professional cleaning—your dentist or a hygienist? Given a choice, our answer is the hygienist. Dental hygienists are prevention specialists with an education in dental hygiene that ranges from two to four years. A dentist's training is focused on restoring teeth and treating advanced gum and bone disease. Cleaning the gums and teeth is a specific treatment that hygienists do all day long. Today, a state-of-the-art preventive dental practice employs qualified registered dental hygienists to be responsible for your hygiene needs. There are exceptions to every rule, and not every dental office has a dental hygienist. In rural areas, it may be more difficult for a dental practice to hire a hygienist, but in the "big city" that should not be a problem.

After the cleaning, a confident hygienist will hand you a mirror and ask if you have any concerns that you want to discuss before you leave. The hygienist will also want to know how your teeth and gums feel and look to you. If you see any stains, ask the hygienist if they are removable because some stains are and some are not.

Do-It-Yourself Follow-up

Following your hygiene visit, monitor the health of your gums, do a visual exam, and apply the tongue test to your teeth:

- Examine your teeth. Do they look white?

- Run your tongue across your teeth. Do your teeth feel slick and clean to the tongue?

- When you floss at home, does the floss slide easily between your teeth and below the gum line?

- Following your appointment, do your gums feel less and less sensitive each day?

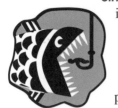

Sink Your Teeth into This: If your gums were bleeding and irritated before your hygiene appointment, closely monitor the condition of your gums during the weeks following your visit. Are your gums in the same state of infection that they were prior to your hygiene visit? Do you continue to experience irritated gums that are red and puffy and bleed?

Each person responds to treatment differently. Depending on body chemistry and the immune system, some individuals take longer to heal. The fact that your gums are still bleeding and irritated one week after your dental hygiene visit may indicate that there is still a deposit problem and a build-up of calculus and tartar, but not necessarily. It can also indicate a medical problem. Call your hygienist and explain your symptoms.

What to Do When There Is a "Cleaning Nightmare"

The "cleaning nightmare" goes like this: You brush and floss and brush and floss, and you still cannot keep the area clean around a filling (or crown or under a bridge), and your gums continue to bleed. No matter how hard you work, the area is resistant to your efforts. At every visit, the hygienist points to the same spot saying this area has an overhang or ledge and needs a more rigorous workout to remove the trapped food and bacteria. What can you do? Ask the dentist or hygienist to point out the troublesome spot on your x-ray (or digital image). One of two things must happen.

THE VIEW FROM THE LEDGE

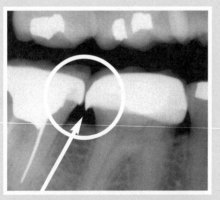

This individual has an overhang at the back of the lower molar. It catches food which can cause decay and gum and bone disease. It also catches and cuts the floss.

When you see the ledge or overhang, you will acquire a better understanding of what you are up against (see the image on the left). You can decide at that point to replace the dental work. Or you can wait another three months and make the decision at your next hygiene visit. Perhaps you feel you haven't worked as hard as you could to keep the area clean. Or maybe you can't afford to replace the work immediately. You can work on the area at home by flossing, brushing, and using an oral irrigator (Water Pik®) several times a day. At your next hygiene appointment, the deciding factor for what to do next will be whether you have been able to keep the area clean and infection-free.

If there is still bleeding, plaque build-up, and gum infection present, you should have the troublesome dental work replaced with a filling, crown, or bridge that can be cleaned more easily and has no offending overhangs or ledges to catch food or floss. Take yourself out of the high-risk category for decay, gum and bone disease, and ultimately tooth loss. Have the repair done.

The Authors' Dental Portraits

A panoramic x-ray is a diagnostic tool for the dentist. It provides both doctor and patient with a view of the teeth, gums, and jaw. The x-ray uncovers a variety of information about your oral health, what dental work has been done in the past, what repairs are necessary, and what to watch for in the future.

After reading the authors' stories, you will understand why individual care and a long-term treatment plan differs from person to person. It also becomes obvious that having your teeth in a state of health and prevention makes brushing, flossing, and going to the dentist a whole lot easier!

VICKI AUDETTE:
The Dental Patient Who Has Many Things Wrong!

In Vicki's case, her x-ray provides a narrative of dental tales and woes. In childhood, Vicki did not receive consistent and preventive dental care. This was not unusual behavior during the 1950s. At that time, dentists were not practicing preventive dentistry, and going to the dentist was a priority only when something was wrong. What dental work Vicki *did* receive was frightening. She lost six out of eight molars (not counting her missing wisdom teeth) and four of those were pulled during grade school. This accounts for the large amount of bone loss where she is missing teeth. As an adult, Vicki hated going to the dentist. She lost more teeth, had infected teeth, and made several uninformed dental decisions.

Today, she is at high risk for tooth loss in three ways—decay, gum disease, and a compromised bite due to her missing teeth. Vicki must jump tremendous hygiene hurdles every day. A large area of her mouth is extremely difficult to clean. Her old fillings, crowns, and bridges trap food and harbor bacteria. Her crowded lower teeth make it tough for her to floss effectively, so she battles with gingivitis. Vicki needs a lot of dental work and has many hygiene goals to achieve before she can reach a comfortable state of prevention.

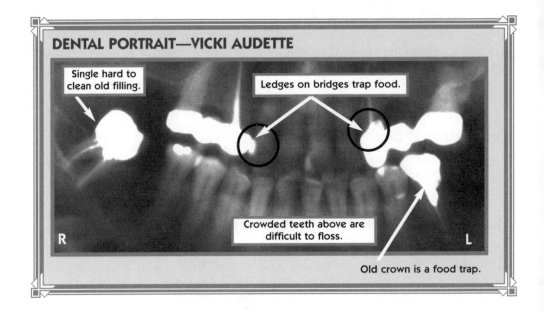

DENTAL PORTRAIT—VICKI AUDETTE

Single hard to clean old filling.

Ledges on bridges trap food.

Crowded teeth above are difficult to floss.

R

L

Old crown is a food trap.

Vicki's Short-term Dental Plan

✔ The large amalgam filling on the single back tooth (see x-ray [R] above) must be replaced with a fixed bridge to allow more biting surface.

✔ The upper [L] bridge has a ledge and must be replaced. Vicki is not an implant candidate because of possible sinus involvement.

✔ The upper [R] bridge is more than 25 years old. It served Vicki well, but it poses a cleaning problem. It is time for retirement. She will need to get a new bridge with an extension which will increase the biting surface.

✔ The old crown and old filling on the lower teeth are both food traps and need to be replaced.

Vicki's Long-term Dental Plan

✔ Possibly minor orthodontics to straighten lower teeth.

✔ Veneers to cosmetically restore her upper front teeth.

When she completes both her short-term and long-term treatment plans, Vicki will have teeth that are easy to clean, a stable bite, and a brighter, more youthful smile.

Pointers and Coaching from Vicki's Hygienist

Vicki's daily mouth care routine has improved in the past year. She now flosses twice a day and brushes both morning and night. Her goal is to reach the ultimate five-times-a-day brushing and flossing routine. Her professional cleaning visits are every three months. And, she can't put off these appointments or she risks serious gum and bone infection.

In reviewing Vicki's past medical history, it appears that her immune system has been overworked and stressed. Her medical background includes double carotid artery surgery at age 47. Her surgery and her inherited high cholesterol have placed her in a compromised cardiovascular health category. So, it is vital that she keep her gums infection-free. To stay healthy, Vicki *must* complete her short-term dental plan.

Vicki also had to alter certain lifestyle habits. For example, she quit smoking several years before we met, but she was in the habit of chewing sugarless gum constantly. Due to her missing teeth and compromised bite, the constant chewing put too much stress on her teeth and bite. It took several months for her to completely quit this habit—but she did it.

Mouth Care Workouts

◆ Vicki switched from a traditional toothbrush to an electric toothbrush and it made a positive difference in her brushing habits, which showed up in her next cleaning visit. She now brushes more often and for a longer period of time.

◆ It took several demonstrations of flossing and floss threader techniques and watching Vicki handle the floss, before she was able to do it effectively under her bridges and between her crowded teeth.

◆ At the point when Vicki had increased her brushing and flossing routine to twice a day, her dental team advised her to add an oral irrigation device to her nightly mouth care routine.

Victoria's Secrets?

"My gums are sensitive, so I prefer Oxygene® Toothpaste and Oxyfresh® mouth rinse, which I buy at my dentist's office. For cleaning under my bridges I like ORAL-B's SuperFloss.®"

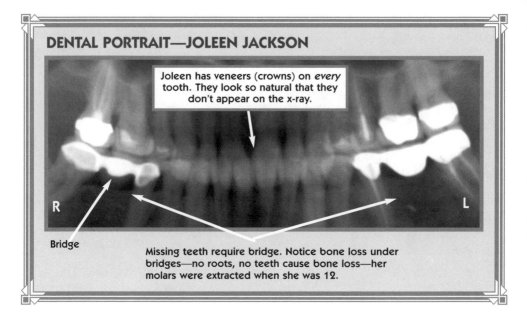

DENTAL PORTRAIT—JOLEEN JACKSON

Joleen has veneers (crowns) on *every* tooth. They look so natural that they don't appear on the x-ray.

R

L

Bridge

Missing teeth require bridge. Notice bone loss under bridges—no roots, no teeth cause bone loss—her molars were extracted when she was 12.

JOLEEN JACKSON
The Dental Patient Who Does It All Right!

Joleen has traveled the "bumpy dental road" that Vicki is presently on. Her childhood dental history was similar to Vicki's. At age seven, Joleen's lower, six-year molars were removed, and while in the sixth grade, she had decay in every molar. Joleen is typical of many baby boomers between the ages of 40 and 60, whose teeth have been filled and re-filled several times. In her case, she had large amalgam fillings. Her dental options were limited. She could wait until most of the teeth were broken down and require extraction. Or she could make an investment in her teeth and save them. Nine years ago, Joleen completed all her dental repairs and cosmetic restorations. Today her dental journey is smooth sailing. Her teeth and gums are in a healthy, prevention state. Her hygiene routine includes a professional cleaning every six months and visits to see the dentist twice a year.

Daily Prevention Routine

Joleen has a sizable investment of time and money in her mouth. She has crowns on every tooth, and as a result, she is super-diligent about her daily mouth care. She brushes and flosses after every meal. (She is not shy; she will floss anywhere!) She always carries a traditional toothbrush, floss, and floss threaders in her purse. At home, she uses an electric toothbrush. At night, she adds an oral irrigator to her nightly brushing and flossing routine to rinse under her bridges. Because she grinds her teeth, she wears a night guard to bed.

Joleen, the Makeover Queen

"At night, I rub fluoride gel along the gum line. Because I grind my teeth, they are very sensitive and the gel helps. Ask your hygienist if this will work for you. Even though I floss many, many times a day—I still depend on my Water Pic® at night to do a thorough job."

Dr. Mac Lee:
The Dentist Who Is Also a Lucky Dental Patient

As a third-generation dentist, Mac Lee is the lucky one. He grew up in a family who knew how to take care of teeth. He is missing only his wisdom teeth. But being a child of the '50s, he also received the dentistry of that time. While in the fourth grade, he broke a tooth down to the gum line. His father performed a root canal (his first one), practicing on Mac's tooth. It is still going strong today. Mac is at very low risk for decay or gum disease and his bite is perfect. He has had his large amalgam fillings replaced by crowns and he had some cosmetic dentistry done. His mouth is in a prevention state and he doesn't have to work very hard to keep it that way. He does wish, however, that his teeth were whiter.

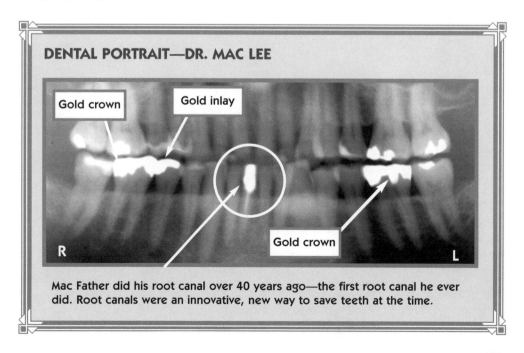

DENTAL PORTRAIT—DR. MAC LEE

Gold crown

Gold inlay

Gold crown

R   L

Mac Father did his root canal over 40 years ago—the first root canal he ever did. Root canals were an innovative, new way to save teeth at the time.

A Dental Wish List

Four years ago, Dr. Buddy Lee (Mac's brother) put veneers on his four front teeth and matched the color perfectly to his natural teeth. Today, people are going whiter and brighter than their natural teeth. Mac wants to have his front teeth redone with a whiter more youthful smile.

Daily Prevention Routine

He uses a traditional toothbrush and floss in the shower every morning. At night, he uses an electric toothbrush and floss before bed.

Lee's General Product Advice

"My favorite is a Rota-Point® floss pick that I use several times throughout the day. I especially like it because it gives me the freedom to do more than one thing at a time."

TOOTH OR CONSEQUENCES
The Daily Mouth Care Routine

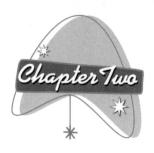

Sixty-five years ago, folks didn't put too much thought into selecting a toothbrush because there was only one style available—a standard model with wild boar bristles. The main flossing tool for a long time was a toothpick, and baking soda served as toothpaste. Today, the mouth care selections may cover an entire aisle in the supermarket. Floss fills shelf space and shoppers can take their pick of waxed, unwaxed, flavored, or unflavored. Power-assisted and traditional toothbrushes are displayed next to a dizzying array of toothpastes that come in a variety of flavors with a host of different cleaning ingredients, including a favorite blast from the past—baking soda.

It is a new age for mouth care and there are a lot of user-friendly tools at your fingertips. The job of removing food and plaque from all the surfaces of the teeth and below the gum line has become more sophisticated as different tools for home use are assigned to do specific tasks. In this chapter, our focus is totally on you and your mouth care fitness. We give you ways to increase and expand your brushing and flossing routine. To do a good job, you need the right tools, the right technique (that's where your personal coach comes in handy), and a little bit of time and personal effort.

Aim for the Right Targets

Certain mouth care tools are designed to clean specific surfaces on your teeth and below your gums. Today, there are so many different cleaning tools to choose from. To avoid any confusion, we have matched the specific cleaning areas of your mouth with the necessary cleaning tools it takes to do a good job. The better you adapt to each tool, the better the job you will do and the more frequently you will do it. And the right tool can take the bite out of brushing. For example, people who use electric toothbrushes like the convenience. While brushing, they can move around the house, watch TV, go help the kids, or read the newspaper.

You have two target areas to clean. Target One is your gums and Target Two is your teeth. Each target is cared for and cleaned in a different way, but the goal is the same—to keep your gums and teeth healthy.

Target One—The Gums

It is not difficult to clean your gums. There are many products that will make the job of removing plaque and trapped food from between the teeth and below the gum line easy.

The Basic Cleaning Tools Include:

☑ **FLOSS** —The styles and variety of dental floss available are waxed, unwaxed, flavored, unflavored, wide, and narrow. Our personal preference is a wide, flat, waxed floss that is also flavored and nicely hugs the tooth while cleaning in between the teeth and under the gums. Some wide, flat, waxed flosses include Oral-B Satinfloss®, Glide by Gore® and Reach® from Johnson and Johnson.

☑ **WOOD OR PLASTIC TOOTHPICKS** —Plastic picks such as Rota-point® are available through dental offices. Interdental cleaners and wood picks such as Stimudent® by Johnson and Johnson are available in stores. These are helpful tools to add to your flossing routine. You can dislodge plaque and massage your gums with the toothpick while working at the computer, watching TV, or reading a book.

Cleaning Tools to Add to Your Target One Routine:

☑ **TINY BRUSH**—A tiny brush is a tool that fits into the end of a handle and is used to clean and massage the gums. These little brushes work well for people with wide spaces between their teeth or people with braces, fixed bridges, or dental implants. Butler and Oral-B brands are available in stores.

☑ **GUM STIMULATOR**—A gum stimulator is a tool with a rubber tip that sits on the end of a handle. You rub the tip along your gum line and it massages and stimulates the gums. Oral-B and Butler have gum stimulators available in stores. Or ask your hygienist for more details.

✓ **FLOSS THREADER**—This tool holds a special floss with a stiff end that gets pulled under a fixed bridge or braces in order to reach and clean areas that your toothbrush can't clean. Oral-B SuperFloss® or Glide® Threader Floss is available in stores.

✓ **FLOSS HOLDERS**—When traditional floss is too difficult to hold and manipulate or an area is hard to reach, a floss holder is a great assistant. The tool holds the floss for you. Floss holders are also recommended when a physical limitation interferes with your flossing.

✓ **ORAL IRRIGATION**—This device is a rinsing tool that forces water, medication, or some type of solution in a steady stream below the gum line. The fluid can penetrate a gum pocket three millimeters deep. This device is essential for people with braces, gum disease, old dental work, or sensitive teeth. The device assists in getting rid of any stubborn food and plaque that may still be lodged after flossing and brushing. Products include Water Pik® by Teledyne or Braun Oral-B OXYJET®. Both are available through your dentist or in stores.

NOTE: If for any reason you are unable to use traditional flossing methods, ask your dental hygienist whether he or she can suggest other options including an electric interdental cleaning device.

Flossing: The Thing We Love to Hate

Most people will admit that they don't floss their teeth on a daily basis. We know because we ask. Yet, people feel guilty because they don't floss often enough. On the top 10 list of hygiene habits people hate to do, flossing ranks very high. Nobody knows for sure why people hate to floss. Complaints we often hear include: it is too tedious; it's too difficult to do; and it hurts. These objections can all be overcome with the help of a good hygienist.

On the flip side, people who do floss daily say they would never turn the clock back and go a day without flossing. We can say with certainty that the more often you floss, the bet-

---

MOUTH RINSE: ARE YOU MASKING POTENTIAL PROBLEMS?

Are you using a mouth rinse on a daily basis to cover a bad odor in your mouth? If the answer is yes, you could be masking a larger problem. Chronic bad breath can be a symptom of a more serious problem such as gum disease, sinus problems, or gastrointestinal disorders. Don't go for a quick, temporary fix. Go for a long-term solution. Ask your dentist or hygienist about the odor in your mouth. If necessary, your dental professional can recommend an ADA-approved mouth rinse.

WHAT DOES THE ADA SEAL OF APPROVAL MEAN?

For more than 100 years, consumers and dentists have relied on the American Dental Association's Seal of Approval as a symbol that a dental care product is safe and effective. Companies and manufacturers of dental care products voluntarily have their products evaluated and tested, so they can receive and market their products with the ADA Seal of Approval. Look for the ADA Seal of Approval when buying toothpaste, mouth rinses, floss, electric toothbrushes, and oral irrigators.

ter the odds that it will become a habit. And when it's a habit, you won't be able to tolerate it when you can't floss.

Author Vicki Audette is a good example of how this works in real life. Initially, she resisted flossing on a daily basis. She averaged about three times a week. After a comprehensive dental examination, she understood her cleaning challenges and made it a goal to floss once a day. It took six months before she moved herself to flossing twice a day. Today, she loves the fact that she is in the habit of doing the thing she used to hate—flossing.

Why Floss Is Your Friend

Make friends with your floss. It may become the next fountain of youth. In his book *Real Age: Are You as Young as You Can Be?*, author Dr. Michael F. Roizen says that flossing your teeth regularly can make your "Real Age" as much as 6.4 years younger. To prevent unnecessary aging, he recommends that we do the things that we already know we should be doing including brushing our teeth with fluoride and going to the dentist at least once (preferably twice) a year. He says "keep flossing because each time you floss you are making yourself younger."

A thorough tooth brushing is very important, but brushing cannot and will not get the plaque that gets between your teeth and below your gums. Forty percent of the cleaning work on your teeth and gums is done when you floss. An enduring misconception that surrounds floss is that its main purpose is to remove uncomfortable pieces of food stuck between the teeth. But it really has a more important purpose. Floss cleans in between each tooth and below the gum line. It removes trapped food and eliminates possible breeding areas for bacteria.

Floss or Die?

The more you floss, the less your chances of developing gum and bone disease. Research has linked gum disease to other systemic diseases, and studies suggest that gum disease may pose a significant health risk. We know for certain, however, that gum and bone disease, when left untreated, can cause bone loss and tooth loss. But this can be easily prevented, if you resolve to take three important action steps:

- ✔ Get regular dental check-ups.
- ✔ Get regular professional cleanings.
- ✔ Brush and floss daily.

Get Friendly with Your Floss

The next time you get your teeth cleaned, let your hygienist critique your flossing technique. Ask her to observe while you floss. In the meantime, here are some flossing tips to help you practice:

1. Take about 18 to 24 inches of floss and wrap it around your middle fingers until you have about a two-inch length between them.

2. Curve the floss around each tooth in a "C" shape (see 1) and guide the floss between the teeth. Use an up and down cleaning motion along the sides of the teeth while sliding the floss gently below the gum line (see 2) to remove plaque and food.

3. Bring forward a fresh section of new floss for each tooth. If you have gingivitis, you may get some bleeding when you first start flossing. This can indicate infection, but don't stop flossing. In fact, if you floss more often, the bleeding may stop after a few days. After a week, if the bleeding has not let up, contact your dentist or hygienist.

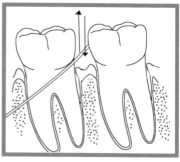

WRONG WAY

FLOSS RIGHT

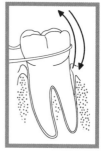

1. RIGHT WAY

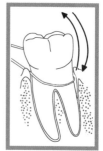

2. RIGHT WAY

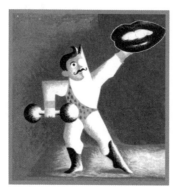

Try This Exercise

We suggest you try this simple exercise. If you are not currently flossing on a regular basis but would like to get started, floss once a day for one month. Then graduate yourself and floss twice a day (morning and night) for another month. If you keep this up for six months, your flossing will become a habit and part of your daily routine. You will love the way your mouth feels. And you can unload all that cumbersome guilt!

Target Two—The Teeth

Concentrate your brushing on the areas of the teeth and gums that you can feel with your tongue including the front and back surfaces of the teeth, the sides and tops of your back molars. And don't forget the tongue itself.

☑ **TOOTHBRUSHES**—The list is long. Many styles, shapes, colors, and features are available. You can find toothbrushes with colorful rubber grip handles or handles that are small, curved, straight, or oversized. And there is least one toothbrush that is specifically made for left-handed folks. The brush itself may be big or small or have uneven bristles that clean hard-to-reach areas or may tilt back to navigate around the teeth. Some brands have color-coded bristles that alert you when it's time to get a new brush.

☑ **POWER-DRIVEN TOOTHBRUSHES**—Name-brand electric toothbrushes will vary in their cleaning movements and added features. Some rotate back and forth; others move up and down. Added features may include two-minute brushing timers and colored bristles to let you know when to replace the brush. Popular

BRIGHT ADVICE ABOUT TOOTHPASTE

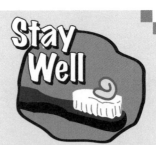

The next time you are browsing the store shelves in search of toothpaste for your kids, choose one that has no sugar or sacchrine. Read the labels:

1. Choose toothpaste that contains fluoride.

2. If you have sensitive teeth, select toothpaste designed for sensitive teeth.

3. Be aware that toothpaste containing baking soda or hydrogen peroxide makes a great cleaning agent, but these ingredients cannot replace fluoride. Select toothpaste that contains all three ingredients. And look for the ADA Seal of Approval because you don't want to make a selection that will be too abrasive.

4. Try changing toothpaste if your gums feel irritated. Tartar control ingredients in toothpaste have been known to irritate gums in some people.

5. Fluoride is an important issue for children and their teeth. Use only a pea-sized amount of toothpaste on your child's toothbrush. It is very important that your child doesn't swallow and ingest fluoride.

brand names are Braun Oral-B® and Sonicare® by Optiva which are available in dental offices and stores. There is also Roto-dent® by Pro-Dentec, which is available only in dental offices.

☑ **TOOTHPASTES**—Toothpaste will vary in flavor and ingredients. Cleaning ingredients will include fluoride, tartar control agents, baking soda, and/or whitening agents. Certain toothpastes, such as the Sensodyne® brand, are for those with sensitive teeth. Read the ingredient labels.

Sink Your Teeth into This: What about fluoride for adults? Sometimes a fluoride toothpaste is not enough (and sometimes, for kids, it is too much). But fluoride can be a therapeutic asset. It can strengthen the teeth and kill the bacteria that cause decay. Your dentist can prescribe gels, tablets, and rinses when necessary.

Brushing: Don't Give Us the Brush-Off!

Your daily brushing habits and techniques will make all the difference in the health of your teeth. During your professional teeth-cleaning appointments, your hygienist should be giving you mouth care advice you can use at home. This includes showing you areas of your mouth where you need to spend extra time or teeth that you may be missing with your toothbrush. If this has not happened, ask your hygienist if there is any place in your mouth that you should be concentrating on during your cleaning routine. Here's a good way to brush your teeth with a traditional toothbrush. You need to spend at least two to three minutes brushing to really make a difference:

BRUSH RIGHT

A
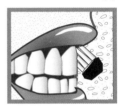

B
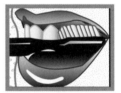

C
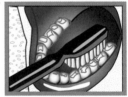

D
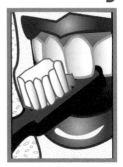

- ◆ Place your brush at a 45-degree angle (A and B) and apply gentle pressure as you move the brush in a short circular motion. The brush should touch both your teeth and your gum line. Avoid using a back and forth motion because it can cause the gums to recede.

- ◆ To brush the back teeth, close your mouth down almost all the way to allow your toothbrush to get behind the back molars. Sometimes this takes practice because your cheek and tongue sets up a natural barrier when you try to get to that particular spot.

- ◆ Be sure to brush the chewing surfaces on the top of your molars (C). Hold the brush flat and move it back and forth.

- ◆ On the inside surfaces (the tongue side) of the front teeth (D), tilt the brush vertically and use gentle up and down strokes with the tip of the toothbrush.

- When you are finished cleaning your teeth, brush your tongue from back to front.

- Rinse your mouth with water. Tap your toothbrush against the sink and wash the bristles thoroughly under water to remove any food or bacteria.

Power-assisted (electric) toothbrushes have come a long way to guide us and make the job of brushing our teeth a whole lot easier. Clinical studies show the electric toothbrush to be superior to traditional toothbrushes. We highly recommend all of the major brands. An electric toothbrush will prove to be a worthwhile investment. They are available through stores and at dental offices. Ask your hygienist for a recommendation.

A Brush with Kindness

Treat your teeth kindly. Brushing not only cleans the front, tops, and back (tongue side) of your teeth and protects them from plaque build-up, it also works to massage your gums and keep them stimulated and healthy. Here's some good advice about brushing: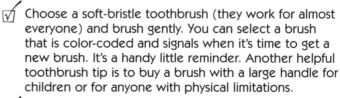

☑ Choose a soft-bristle toothbrush (they work for almost everyone) and brush gently. You can select a brush that is color-coded and signals when it's time to get a new brush. It's a handy little reminder. Another helpful toothbrush tip is to buy a brush with a large handle for children or for anyone with physical limitations.

☑ Use only a pea-size amount of toothpaste (for adults and especially for kids). It is the brushing motion that is cleaning the teeth. The purpose of toothpaste is to apply small amounts of fluoride on the teeth and to make breath fresher.

☑ The next time you brush, time yourself. Brushing works best when you brush for at least two minutes. There are electric toothbrushes that have built-in, two-minute timers.

☑ Add one more brushing to your daily routine. And make sure you always brush before bed. Do it for one month—until it becomes a habit.

☑ If you absolutely can't brush after a meal, vigorously rinse your mouth with water or chew sugarless gum. It helps dislodge unwanted surface food. Stay away from sugared gum. It will only add to the unwanted acids in your mouth. Be aware, however, that a water rinse, mouth rinse, or sugarless gum can not make up for a good brushing.

- ☑ Keep an extra toothbrush and toothpaste at your desk, as well as sugar-free gum.

- ☑ Add power to your mouth care routine. Electric dental tools are a great solution for people who don't have the dexterity or patience to thoroughly brush their teeth.

- ☑ Get rid of your old toothbrush every one to two months. (And replace the brush on your electric toothbrush too!) You can remove more plaque with a toothbrush that is one month old than you can with a brush three months old. As a precaution, replace your brush after you have been sick with a cold or an infection.

- ☑ Never share your toothbrush! Decay and gum infections are transmissible.

- ☑ Drink at least seven glasses of water a day to keep the saliva flowing in your mouth. This is even more important as you get older and your saliva flow is reduced.

PAMPER YOUR GUMS AND CLEAN YOUR DENTURES (AND PARTIAL DENTURES)

The most important reason to clean your dentures and partial dentures each day is to protect your gums from getting irritated by any plaque build-up on the denture (or partial). Cleaning will also help to remove any stains on your dentures.

- ◆ Place the denture in warm (not hot) water or a denture-soaking solution (usually comes in tablet form). Use a denture brush to clean off the plaque.

- ◆ Another cleaning option is an ultrasonic device that mechanically cleans the denture. Ask your dentist for more information.

- ◆ To remove any bad odors on the denture or partial, soak it in a mixture of one teaspoon of baking soda added to eight ounces of water. Soak for at least one hour.

- ◆ When finished with your cleaning routine, give your gums a massage to stimulate the blood circulation. If you have any sores on your gums, contact your dentist.

☑ Keep your brain alive. Try brushing your teeth with the opposite hand. According to author Lawrence Katz, in his book *Keep Your Brain Alive: 83 Neurobic Exercises*, this exercise will stimulate the neuro-pathways in the brain. (Does this mean the more you brush, the smarter you will be?)

☑ And finally, you may want to get yourself a tongue scraper. Designed with rippled edges, tongue scrapers efficiently scrape and clean and do a much better job on your tongue than your toothbrush.

STRAIGHT TEETH ARE EASIER TO CLEAN

Braces work to straighten teeth, not only for appearance purposes, but also to make the teeth easier to clean. Your general dentist, orthodontist or pediatric dentist can give you a cleaning video that describes in great detail the home care techniques for cleaning teeth with braces. One of the most important challenges about wearing braces at any age will be to comply with the cleaning and care routine set by your dentist.

The tool recommendations include:

◆ A floss threader

◆ An ADA-recommended fluoride toothpaste (and maybe in-office treatments)

◆ An irrigation device

WHAT'S YOUR PROBLEM?
HERE ARE YOUR SOLUTIONS!

Mouth Care Workouts Just for You

BAD BREATH

The Problem

The cause of halitosis often originates in the mouth and can be taken care of at home. Bacteria in the mouth causes gases to be released which result in bad breath. Improper cleaning of the teeth, gums, and tongue can be the problem. Be aware however that bad breath can also be caused by a variety of other conditions including gum disease, sinus drainage, and respiratory or gastrointestinal problems.

The Workout Routine

Products available at stores or in dental offices for treating bad breath should be used only as an extension of good mouth care, regular dental check-ups, and professional teeth-cleaning appointments. The bad odor may be due to gum disease and may be coming from periodontal pockets below the gum line. When that is the case, the dentist will diagnose and treat the infection until you are disease-free. We don't recommend masking the bad odor with rinses, mints, or gum in an attempt to eliminate the offending smell without determining the cause. In the majority of cases, bad breath can be easily handled. Brushing your tongue, the inside of your cheeks, and the roof of your mouth in order to remove the offending food particles is also very important.

Recommended Tools

◆ A tongue scraper will go a long way in the fight against bad breath. The tongue is a hot spot for bacterial growth.

Dental Care Options

First and foremost, have the dentist or hygienist check for gum and bone disease. In some cases, periodontal therapy may be necessary. Or the bad odor may be caused by a health problem that requires a physician.

CROOKED OR CROWDED TEETH

The Problem

Tough-to-clean areas in the mouth put you at risk for gum disease and decay. Overlapping teeth easily trap food and sugars. This, in turn, feeds the decay causing bacteria to grow a lot faster and more often than it does on straight teeth.

The Workout Routine

Swishing liquid around in your mouth to clear out food and plaque is not effective on straight teeth if it is your only cleaning method. And for crowded teeth, it is a totally useless exercise. If having crooked or crowded teeth is your dilemma, you don't have the luxury of beginning your mouth care routine at a slow pace. You will have to practice a full dental routine *fast*. Crooked teeth require guerrilla cleaning tactics from the get-go. Frequent daily brushing and flossing is as essential as breathing. So take a deep breath and get started!

Recommended Tools

- Floss, floss, and more floss—Stock up because you will need more floss than the average person. Carry it wherever you go, in your purse, gym bag, or brief case. If you put it in your shower, it will help you remember to floss as part of your morning routine.

- An electric toothbrush.

- An irrigation device—Double up your plaque and food removal efforts along with your regular flossing routine.

Dental Care Options

The only dental option we can suggest is to get your crooked and crowded teeth properly aligned with orthodontics in order to make the teeth and gums easier to clean. Discuss this option with your dentist. If orthodontics is not an option for you, you will have to work twice as hard and brush and floss more often.

DECAY-PRONE TEETH

The Problem

Why are some people more prone to tooth decay than others? Lifestyle habits play a big role in whether you get cavities or not. Also a certain percentage of decay-prone folks harbor an over-population of bacteria in their mouths that causes decay. If you are decay-prone, you become a high-risk dental patient who must alter lifestyle habits and routines.

The Workout Routine

A decay-prone person risks losing all of his or her teeth. So what follows is "must do" advice. You must be aware of what you eat and drink and increase your brushing and flossing routine. Similar advice is given to a heart patient. The heart patient must change his/her eating habits and develop a daily walking routine. However, if you have no regular routine for brushing and flossing your teeth, don't get discouraged. Just start somewhere. The best marathon runners didn't begin by running 10 miles a day. Start slowly and work your way up the hygiene ladder. Brush and floss once a day, before bedtime (to prevent overnight sugar and acid from eating away your teeth), until it becomes second nature. Then graduate yourself to a twice-a-day brushing and flossing program. In no time, you will be flossing and brushing at least three times a day.

Recommended Tools
- An electric toothbrush (and keep a traditional toothbrush in your purse or briefcase).
- Floss.
- Toothpaste with fluoride.
- An irrigation device that removes food and plaque that can't be reached by your floss or brush.
- Fluoride treatments at home.

Dental Care Options

Your hygienist will design a daily mouth care routine and suggest a list of tools for your mouth that will make your cleanings at home more effective. You need to be monitored every three to six months by the hygienist to be sure that your home care is on target. If you need extra fluoride, the hygienist may recommend a prescription fluoride gel, fluoride trays, or give you a fluoride treatment. If you continue to get decay, ask your dentist about giving you a saliva test to see if you are one of the individuals who harbors the bacteria that causes decay.

DRY MOUTH SYNDROME

The Problem

Saliva is the body's natural way of cleaning your teeth. People with "dry mouth" (reduced saliva) lose this natural process and become susceptible to the build-up of plaque, which can lead to rampant decay. If you are taking medication, ask your physician if dry mouth is a side effect.

The Workout Routine

Sip water frequently throughout the day (at least eight glasses). Avoid mints, sweets, and sodas that will promote decay. Frequent flossing and brushing every day is essential. And make frequent visits to your hygienist (as often as one- to three-month intervals) for professional cleanings, monitoring for decay, and mouth care fitness advice.

Recommended Tools

- ◆ An electric toothbrush is mandatory.
- ◆ Frequent flossing.
- ◆ Over-the-counter saliva replacement products.

Dental Care Options

The dentist may prescribe fluoride treatments and frequent hygiene check-ups and may discuss saliva replacement products.

TEETH WITH LARGE FILLINGS

The Problem

Large fillings can become food traps and harbor the sugar and acids that increase the number of bacteria that cause decay.

The Workout Routine

The main workout goal is to properly clean between the teeth where the large fillings are located. If you have large fillings, you must brush and floss more frequently. Let your hygienist work as your personal trainer to give you suggestions for thoroughly cleaning areas with large fillings. Discuss any cleaning difficulties you may have.

Recommended Tools

- ◆ Floss—If you have difficulty with floss, try a floss holder. It may make the job easier.
- ◆ An irrigation device will increase your flossing effectiveness.

Dental Care Options

If the filling is very large and/or chipped, it may be impossible to keep clean. When that is the case, it may be necessary to remove the filling and replace it with a new filling or get the tooth crowned. Your dentist will discuss your dental repair options. We suggest you do whatever it takes to make the tooth cleansible.

FIXED BRIDGES OR MULTIPLE DENTAL IMPLANTS

The Problem

Anyone with bridges or implants (the kind that are joined together) can testify about the special challenges of flossing. For a fixed bridge, it is essential that you clean *underneath* the artificial teeth. That is where food can get trapped and become a breeding area for plaque and bacteria.

The Workout Routine

Floss under the bridge to eliminate food and plaque. If you don't clean that area, the tissue can swell and eventually you can lose the bridge because of infection.

Recommended Tools

- ◆ A floss threader—Ask your hygienist to show you how to clean under the bridge.

- ◆ An irrigation device.

- ◆ Small brushes for cleaning around the implant—Ask your hygienist about Butler's Flossbrush® system.

Dental Care Options

If your hygienist says you've got red, puffy, or bleeding gums because your fixed bridge is trapping food, you may eventually need to replace the bridge, especially if the infection is persistent. Ask your hygienist for hands-on, step-by-step cleaning techniques and instructions. The dentist may also recommend that you get tissue removed from around the bridge in order to make that area of your mouth more cleansible.

GINGIVITIS

The Problem

Look for signs of bleeding. Your toothbrush or floss may appear pink or red. Pull your bottom lip down and examine your gums. Do they look red or puffy? Gingivitis and gum infection will not heal themselves. These conditions require a diagnosis and a treatment plan from a dental professional. If you see signs or have symptoms of gingivitis or gum disease, be sure to contact your dentist or hygienist as quickly as possible.

The Workout Routine

"If it bleeds, it needs." That's a phrase dental folks often use. It means that bleeding gums are not normal. Bleeding can signal that something needs to be done. Gingivitis requires a workout routine that also cleans below the gum line. The bleeding may also indicate that the immune system may be involved and there may be damage to the protective, connective tissue that surrounds the tooth. Frequent, daily flossing is necessary, along with frequent monitoring by your hygienist. She or he will provide step-by-step coaching and advise you concerning your brushing and flossing techniques. Brush your gums as well as your teeth and gently massage your gums with a toothbrush or a rubber-tipped stimulator. It won't feel comfortable at first, but keep at it. The healthier your gums get, the better they will feel. And by that time, you will have developed a good brushing and flossing routine.

Recommended Tools

◆ Floss and floss picks—To encourage its use, make sure floss is strategically located both at home and at work. Place floss near the phone, in the shower, in a make-up case, or on your desk.

◆ An electric toothbrush for home use.

◆ A traditional toothbrush for easy "take along" use during the day, while at work or school.

◆ A rubber-tipped gum stimulator.

Dental Care Options

The frequency of your hygiene visits will be based on your individual needs and will be determined by your dentist. Your dentist may also prescribe a professional mouth rinse such as *chlorhexidine*.

MODERATE TO ADVANCED GUM AND BONE DISEASE

The Problem

Moderate to advanced gum and bone disease is the leading cause of tooth loss. Often there is no pain until the later stages. Look for signs of bleeding, bad breath, and low energy (see Section II for more in-depth information).

The Workout Routine

Run, don't walk, to your dentist if there is serious gum and bone disease. When gum disease is present, your mouth care routine must be accelerated. Get on the brushing and flossing fast track. Concentrate your efforts below the gum line where periodontal pockets are harboring bacteria.

Recommended Tools

◆ Double the number of times you floss each day.

◆ An electric toothbrush is essential.

◆ An irrigation device to increase the effectiveness of eliminating any trapped food and plaque.

Dental Care Options

Keep in close contact with your hygienist. Regular visits at short intervals are a must to ensure that your home brushing and flossing is on target. Periodontal surgery to lower the gum line in order to clean more thoroughly may be a necessary treatment after deep scaling and root planing procedures have been performed.

SENSITIVE TEETH

The Problem

The problem of sensitive teeth is one of the mysteries in dentistry. The cause is not always known. Sensitivity can be due to teeth not fitting together properly, a build-up of plaque, lifestyle habits, or "dentin hypersensitivity." That's when the enamel of your teeth is worn away, which leaves the dentin exposed and causes sensitivity to hot or cold food and drinks.

WAS IT SOMETHING I ATE?

Sensitive teeth can be caused by genetic and/or lifestyle habits. In other words, you can inherit sensitive teeth, or you may be doing something to aggravate the problem.

◆ Do cut back on high acid foods and juices.

◆ Don't brush teeth aggressively. A gentle brushing is all that is needed.

◆ Do use a soft toothbrush.

◆ Don't use a tartar-control toothpaste. The active ingredient may irritate your sensitivity problem.

◆ Don't use chewing tobacco or smoke cigarettes (or cigars).

If nothing helps, turn to your dentist and hygienist and discuss possible dental options.

Unfortunately, the sensitivity issue can create a vicious cycle. When teeth are sensitive, people often don't feel like brushing and flossing because it hurts. But if you don't brush and floss, the plaque that causes the sensitivity builds up and the sensitivity continues. The answer? Continue to brush and floss.

The Workout Routine

If your teeth are sensitive, develop a mouth care routine to fit the problem. Talk to your hygienist about your sensitive teeth. Inquire about changing some of your mouth care tools and techniques. Maintain a daily mouth fitness regimen—brushing thoroughly, flossing, and visiting your dentist and hygienist regularly.

Recommended Tools

◆ A soft toothbrush.

◆ Over-the-counter toothpaste designed for sensitive teeth (use only a small amount of paste). If your regular toothpaste has a tartar control ingredient, it may help to switch to a brand without it.

◆ An irrigation device that uses warm water (or salt water).

◆ Fluoride gel treatments rubbed along the gum line at night may help with the sensitivity.

Dental Care Options

If you cannot get relief, make an appointment with your dentist. He or she may prescribe additional fluoride treatments (or fluoride trays for home use). The dentist may also apply sealants to the sensitive teeth.

THE PHYSICALLY CHALLENGED CAN OVERCOME CLEANING HURDLES

When manual dexterity is an issue, special mouth care fitness tools and techniques may help. Ask for the assistance of a hygienist to guide you with your brushing and flossing techniques. He or she can also help you locate special tools. A once-a-month professional cleaning will do wonders and help to prevent decay and gum disease.

Recommended Tools:

◆ An electric toothbrush. Let the brush do the work for you.

◆ A traditional toothbrush with a large handle, if an electric toothbrush is not an option.

◆ A floss holder to help with flossing dexterity.

SENIOR MOUTH CARE

The Problem

As the rest of the body ages, so does the mouth. Receding gums (and perhaps gum disease), a reduction in saliva, and an increase in plaque build-up on the teeth all make it harder for some older adults to keep their teeth clean. Old fillings can break down and trap food and bacteria. Cleansibility problems put seniors at risk for tooth decay. The good news is that you can slow down the aging process in your mouth. Changes in lifestyle habits and diet may be necessary (especially if you are sucking on mints or cough drops to relieve dry mouth symptoms). Let your dentist and hygienist run interference for you. Early detection of decay or gum disease will help ward off large (and costly) dental repairs.

The Workout Routine

Steer clear of sticky foods, dried fruit, juice with high sugar content, and candy and sweets (mints, cough drops). Drink eight glasses of water daily and eat foods high in fiber to help increase your saliva flow. Get at least two professional teeth-cleanings annually—more often, if necessary.

Recommended Tools

- An ADA-recommended fluoride toothpaste.

- An electric toothbrush to make your cleaning routine a lot easier. Also ask your hygienist for recommendations on other mouth care tools.

- Fluoride tables may be necessary. Ask your dentist.

Dental Care Options

Routinely visit your dentist more often to monitor the health of your mouth and gums and to screen for signs of oral cancer. Dental problems such as missing teeth, ill-fitting dentures or bridges, and/or gum disease will not only make you look older faster but will threaten your overall health. Get any necessary dental repairs completed. Your dentist will have some answers and options to help you keep your teeth and gums healthy.

And Finally . . .

10 THINGS TO DO *RIGHT NOW* TO KEEP YOUR SMILE HEALTHY AND MAKE YOU LOOK 10 YEARS YOUNGER, 10 YEARS FROM NOW!

- Learn to manage stress and you can add years to your life. Less stress is also healthier for your gums.

- Ask your hygienist to coach you on your brushing and flossing routine and to recommend the correct products for your teeth and gums.

- Brush your teeth for at least two minutes twice a day, using a soft traditional or electric toothbrush.

- Floss, floss, floss daily and you'll keep yourself (and your teeth) young.

- Get regular dental check-ups and professional teeth-cleanings twice a year (or at least once a year).

- If your teeth are crooked or crowded, discuss with your dentist the prospect of getting them straightened.

- If you grind or clench your teeth, your dentist may recommend a night guard to protect your teeth from wear and tear.

- If you have old, large fillings or fixed bridges with ledges that make it tough to clean, talk to your dentist and hygienist about the benefits and options for getting old dental repairs replaced.

- Avoid decay. Stop sipping sodas throughout the day or sucking on mints or cough drops (especially while in bed at night).

- *QUIT SMOKING* (or using *any* tobacco products). Contact The Cancer Society or The American Lung Association in your area to find a good "quit smoking" program.

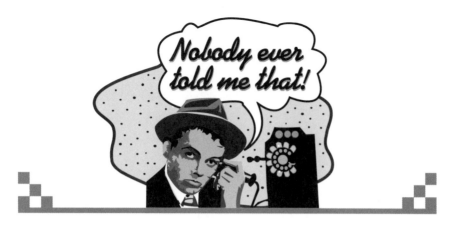

■ Your hygienist is a dental prevention specialist who can act as your brushing and flossing trainer. If you get tied up in your floss, ask your hygienist to observe your flossing technique at your next visit and get some pointers from a pro.

■ Potentially life-threatening signs and symptoms of disease can appear first in the mouth and can be detected at an early stage during a dental examination or a hygiene visit.

■ If you are afraid to get your teeth professionally cleaned because it may hurt, don't worry. Two pain-relieving solutions are available. A special numbing mouth rinse can be used before the cleaning starts. Or you can ask to receive nitrous oxide during your cleaning.

■ If your gums are bleeding and irritated before your hygiene appointment, closely monitor the condition of your gums for a week following your visit. Call your hygienist if your gums continue to bleed and feel irritated.

■ You have two target areas to clean in your mouth. Target One is your gums and Target Two is your teeth.

■ Certain mouth care tools are designed to clean specific surfaces. Floss goes between the teeth and below the gum line. Your toothbrush does the surfaces of the teeth and your tongue (or use a tongue scraper).

■ What the heck is an oral irrigator? A handy device that rinses under fixed bridges and below the gum line. It's a good thing to get if you have problems with gingivitis or gum disease.

■ Mouth rinses can be a problem if they are masking a problem. Ask your dentist or hygienist about chronic bad breath. It may be a sign of gum disease.

■ Get rid of old fillings or any old dental repair that makes it impossible to clean your teeth. Ask your hygienist or dentist for advice.

■ Flossing your teeth every day will help you look 6.4 years younger than your "Real Age." Read all about it in Dr. Michael Roizen's book, *Real Age*.

Who Is a Dental Specialist?

All dental specialties require two or more academic years beyond graduation from dental school. The American Dental Association (ADA) recognizes the following dental specialists:

Endodontists

Diagnose and treat diseases and injuries to the tooth's pulp and the tissues surrounding the root of the tooth.

Oral and Maxillofacial Surgeons

Diagnose and surgically treat diseases, injuries and abnormalities of the hard and soft tissues of the neck, face, head, and jaws. This includes the repair and restoration of oral tissue and supporting structures. They also do surgical procedures such as dental implants, extractions, and tissue and bone grafts.

Orthodontists

Diagnose and treat problems of occlusion (bite) and malformations of the jaws by repositioning the teeth and facial bones using various appliances to restore normal function and appearance.

Pediatric Dentists (Pedodontists)

Specialize in treating the dental needs of children from birth through adolescence.

Periodontists

Prevent, diagnose, and treat periodontal disease and surgically place dental implants.

Prosthodontists

In difficult dental cases, replace missing teeth with a variety of prosthesis such as fixed bridges, dental implants, and partial dentures.

I'm Still Confused, Doc!

Q. *When I get a tooth crowned, does it mean that I never again have to worry about decay?*

A. No. The crown itself will not decay but the portion of the tooth that is not covered by the crown will. To keep the uncovered tooth healthy, use a soft toothbrush and start brushing by pushing upward from the gums to the top of the crown. And of course it goes without saying—floss.

Q. *My dentist found a cavity in a tooth that did not bother me. It has been sensitive to both hot and cold ever since she put the new filling in. What is going on?*

A. There are several possible scenarios:

1) It is possible that the decay went so deep that it was already in the nerve and may need a root canal.

2) The large filling could have traumatized the tooth.

3) If the new filling is too high, the excessive biting pressure may bruise the tooth.

4) In some instances, the filling can leak.

Q. *Why can't the dentist just fill my tooth rather than do a crown?*

A. When the hole left by decay is so large that it weakens the tooth, the tooth needs support from the crown.

Q. *What can be done to make my dental visits less stressful?*

A. The more frequent your visits, the more comfortable you will become. Communication with the dentist and dental team is also important. Talk about what stresses you the most and ask what is available to help you get through feeling anxious. The dentist and dental team should explain how you can be in control during your dental appointments.

Q. *If I had it to do over again, I would get all my teeth fixed in one visit instead of one tooth at a time. Is that possible to do?*

A. Yes, unless your dental problems are too complicated. If your time is short and your schedule is hectic, ask your dentist if a one-stop dental visit is possible.

Q. *Why do I have to have another filling (or crown or partial denture)? It seems that I have to do this often.*

A. It may be that your lifestyle habits are causing decay. An honest, personal review will help. Ask yourself: Are you eating sugar at bedtime and not brushing your teeth? Do you brush and floss twice a day? Are you chewing tobacco? Do you sip colas all day long? Another possibility is that you have never had a comprehensive dental exam. As a result, you were never given a full treatment plan. Or, the dentist did not tell you in the beginning that you would need more dental work.

Q. *My wife says she can't stand my snoring any longer. Can a dentist help me with this?*

A. Sleep apnea must first be ruled out. Then ask your dentist about anti-snoring devices which can help some snoring problems. These dental appliances look a lot like a child's retainer from the orthodontist. The devices help keep the back of the throat open which prevents snoring. It is always best however, to find a dentist who works closely with a physician who has special knowledge of sleep disorders.

Q. *I had a crown replaced and I don't understand why we couldn't just use my old crown? Was my dentist just trying to make extra money on me?*

A. Crowns are very precise restorations. Once the tooth or the crown has been altered by decay or breakage, the crown no longer fits properly. Trying to make it fit will result in grooves or ledges in the junction area of the tooth and crown. This can lead to gum disease and decay because the area will not be cleansible.

Q. *I have dry mouth and I rely on cough drops. I keep a supply next to my bed, in my pockets, and in my desk. Pretty much wherever I go, the cough drops go. Is there any problem with that?*

A. Never keep cough drops or mints near on your bedside table because it is too tempting to eat them before going to bed (or reach for them in the middle of the night). They are both full of sugar. The sugar will lie next to your gums and teeth and cause rampant decay. Severe decay can happen in a matter of days or weeks. This is the type of habit that causes decay at the gum line and attacks all teeth, even the ones with crowns.

Q. *I sip soft drinks all day long. I've heard that may be the reason I have so much decay. What do you think?*

A. There is no question that sodas are causing your decay because having small amounts of sugar in your mouth over long periods of time can be a very serious problem. It doesn't make any difference where the sugar comes from, whether from cough drops or sipping on a soft drink throughout the day. These sugars make a perfect environment for bacteria to cause decay. This habit of sipping drinks is one of the most devastating things that you can do to teeth. You are being hit with a double whammy because the soda also contains acid, and this is doing as much dental damage as the sugar.

Q. *I worry about the spread of disease every time I go to a hospital or doctor's office. How do I know if my dentist is sterilizing properly?*

A. Just ask: "Do you sterilize your equipment with an autoclave using both heat and pressure or with chemicals?" The American Dental Association guidelines recommend that all instruments be autoclaved between patients or be disposed of. This will prevent infection from being transmitted. Chemicals alone are not as effective.

Q. *I have high blood pressure and I am on medication for this condition. Can the medication harm my gums or teeth?*

A. Yes. There are many medications that can cause serious problems for the mouth. Blood pressure medicine can have two negative effects. It can decrease the saliva flow which allows more decay-causing bacteria to grow. It can also cause the gum tissues to swell, which may increase the chances of getting gum disease.

Q. *I have a question concerning dental care while breast-feeding. I have a tooth that has a cracked filling which makes it temperature sensitive and difficult to chew on that side of the mouth. Will it harm the baby if I continue to breast-feed? Also, if I do get the filling fixed will I need to discontinue breast-feeding for any length of time because of medications that are used in numbing the area.*

A. The answer to both questions is no.

Q. *My daughter has been diagnosed with TMD. The disk is out of place, in front of the joint. As a result, it interferes with the opening and closing of her mouth. The oral surgeon is suggesting that she wear a splint for two weeks. Is this reasonable? If this does not work, he recommends surgery. What is the treatment of choice?*

A. Because of its non-invasive nature, a splint is the treatment of choice. Often the result is good. The symptoms will reflect the need for more extensive treatment (i.e., surgery). Surgery should only be a last resort.

Q. *What can I do about my bad breath? I suck mints and clean my teeth often?*

A. Check with your doctor for any underlying medical cause such as a gastric problem or sinus drainage. If the odor is really coming from your mouth, our advice is to get a comprehensive dental exam that looks at both the teeth and gums. Brush your teeth twice a day, floss them every day, and brush or scrape your tongue. This is the most effective way of guarding against bad breath (when there's no other medical reason that is causing the odor). Ask your dentist about breath control products. If you must have something in your mouth, suck on mints that are sugar-free.

Q. *What is the difference between plaque and tartar? Also, when I see the hygienist, what is she scraping off my teeth? I brush, floss, and use a water pick daily. There shouldn't be anything to scrape off my teeth.*

A. Plaque is a soft deposit of bacteria that grows on the teeth and can be removed easily by brushing. When the plaque has calcified (hardened), it becomes tartar. Within days, plaque that is undisturbed by brushing or flossing (usually in the hard-to-reach areas of the mouth) has to be scraped off by a dental professional.

Q. *What causes canker sores?*

A. The exact cause is unknown. Current theories point to an auto-immune disorder. It is also believed that certain factors may initiate the chain of events leading to a canker sore. These factors include sensitivity to certain foods, certain ingredients in toothpaste, stress, and trauma to the lining of the mouth.

Q. *I thought I was too old to get decay. Is this true or not?*

A. No. Decay can destroy your teeth at any age.

Q. *Am I too old to get braces?*

A. No. Teeth can be moved at all ages. If you want straight teeth, ask your dentist about your options.

Q. *Drill-less, pain-free dentistry? What is it all about?*

A. There are two different techniques for removing decay and tooth structure without using the normal drill. One is an air abrasion technique that works like a miniature sand blaster; the second is laser. Both of them work very well for what they were designed to do—remove very small decay at the very beginning stage. This means that only a limited number of people—those with very small decay that is caught right away can get "drill-less dentistry." For these people, this is a bonus because these two different techniques do not have the traditional noise of the drill, which so many people dislike. And, there is usually no discomfort for the patient with either of these techniques.

Q. *My wife heard that there is a new way to find decay. Is this true?*

A. Modern technology has opened up a new way of going beyond early detection of decay and stopping it before it even begins. We now have magnification and special decay-detecting staining dyes that allow us to see the signs of decay just as it is beginning. We have new technology that can remove small amounts of decay without causing trauma to the tooth. And new plastic filling materials are able to flow down into the narrow holes left by the decay. A special light hardens the liquid plastic and seals off the tooth. The technology of dentistry is moving into the next century with promising new advances and more to come.

Glossary

ABSCESS
A mass of infection in either teeth or bone that sometimes (but not always) is associated with pain.

AIR ABRASION
A technology using aluminum oxide under pressure to remove tooth structure and decay. Sometimes referred to as drill-less or shot-less dentistry.

AMALGAM
Dental material used to fill cavities. Commonly called "silver fillings." Usually consists of a mixture of silver and mercury with copper, tin, and zinc particles.

ANTERIOR TEETH
Used to describe the six upper and lower front teeth used as biting and cutting surfaces rather than chewing surfaces.

ANTIBIOTIC
An artificial or natural substance which inhibits or kills bacteria, e.g. penicillin.

ANTIMICROBIAL
A substance or process that destroys or inhibits the growth of bacteria.

APPLIANCE
Any removable dental restoration or orthodontic device.

APHTHOUS STOMATITIS
The medical term given to an outbreak of canker sores. Also called "recurrent aphthous stomatitis" or "aphthous ulcer."

BACTEREMIA
Bacteria in the bloodstream.

BITEWING X-RAY
An x-ray of the crowns of the upper and lower back teeth taken together to view how the teeth fit with one another and to identify possible areas of decay.

BLEACHING
A cosmetic dental procedure to remove stains from teeth and make them whiter.

BONDING
A cosmetic dental procedure in which a tooth-colored plastic is applied with adhesive to change the shape or shade of a tooth.

BRACES
Orthodontic appliances applied to teeth to correct crowding and malocclusion.

BRUXISM
Grinding, clenching, or gnashing of teeth.

CALCULUS	A tenacious, hardened material formed by mineralization (calcification) of dental plaque.
CAP	Another name for a crown.
CARIES	The technical term for cavities or tooth decay. Also called a "cavity."
CEMENTUM	Covers the root of the tooth. Serves as the anchor point for the ligaments that join the tooth to the bony tooth socket. The softest of the tooth structures.
COSMETIC DENTISTRY	A type of dentistry that involves procedures done solely to improve appearance.
CROWN	Portion of tooth covered by enamel. Also refers to a dental restoration shaped like the tooth it covers.
DEBRIDEMENT	Treatment of bacterial infection by removing irritants (bacteria, calculus) from the periodontal pocket in order to allow healing of the adjacent tissues.
DECIDUOUS TEETH	Baby teeth or primary teeth.
DEMINERALIZATION	A loss of mineral from tooth enamel. May appear as a small, white area on the tooth surface.
DENTAL ASSISTANT	A professional who works chair-side with a dentist, setting up equipment for procedures, handing instruments, and carrying out procedures and other general assistance tasks.
DENTAL HYGIENIST	A trained professional who cleans teeth, takes x-rays, carries out preliminary oral examinations, and provides education on oral hygiene. State laws vary as to other tasks a hygienist may perform.
DENTAL RESIN	A plastic filling applied to the tooth.
DENTIN	The main tissue that forms the shape of the tooth. This material exists between the pulp and the enamel and is composed of a series of dentinal tubules stacked on top of each other.

ENAMEL	The hard, mineralized, white material which covers the outside of the tooth.
ERUPTION	When teeth first peek through gums.
EXPLORER	A probe used to detect cavity growth.
EXTRACTION	Removal of a tooth.
FISSURES	Cleft-like grooves in the chewing surface of the back teeth.
FIXED BRIDGE	A prosthesis used to replace one or more missing teeth that is permanently attached at both ends to artificial crowns placed on the remaining teeth.
FLUORIDE	A chemical compound that helps strengthen teeth as well as reduce tooth decay and sensitivity.
FLUOROSIS	Discoloration of the enamel due to too much fluoride ingestion (greater than one part per million), which then enters the bloodstream. Also called "enamel mottling."
GENERAL DENTIST	A dentist educated and trained on all dental procedures, but who does not specialize in only one particular facet of dentistry.
GINGIVAL MARGIN	The area of gingiva that is closest to the tooth surface. Commonly referred to as the "gum line."
GINGIVA	The dense tissue surrounding the teeth and covering the alveolar bone. Commonly referred to as "gums."
GINGIVITIS	Generally refers to an inflammation of the gingiva (gums) and ranges in classification from mild to severe. Symptoms include redness, swelling, bleeding, and tenderness of the gingiva.
HARD PALATE	The bony front portion of the roof of the mouth.
HANDPIECE	The dentist's drill.
HYPERPLASIA	Overgrowth of the gingival tissues. This can continue until a large portion of the teeth is covered by gingival tissue.

HYPERSENSITIVITY	A sharp, sudden, painful reaction when the teeth are exposed to hot, cold, chemical, mechanical, or osmotic (sweet or salt) stimuli.
IMAGERY	A digital, high-tech process for doing an x-ray that uses 90% less radiation. Also called a "digital image."
IMMUNE RESPONSE	The body's natural defense against bacterial assault. The immune response can also destroy alveolar bone in its attempt to destroy bacteria.
IMPACTED TOOTH	A tooth that does not erupt into its normal position but remains fully or partially embedded in the bone.
IMPLANTS (DENTAL)	Replace missing teeth by using a titanium anchor that is implanted into the jaw bone. An artificial tooth (or dentures) is then fitted over the implant.
IMPRESSION	An imprint of some or all of the teeth and gums made in a soft material from which a study cast is made. Used in preparing crowns, bridges, dentures, partial dentures, bleaching trays, and orthodontic treatments.
INTRA-ORAL CAMERA	A small camera used in the mouth for magnification of the teeth and gums and used as a visual aid for the patient. The image is shown on a monitor and can be viewed by both the dentist and the patient.
INTERDENTAL	Between the teeth.
IRRIGATION	Mechanical method of flushing with fluid to disrupt debris and plaque.
JAW DYSFUNCTION	Abnormal operation of the temporomandibular joint (TMJ). A dysfunction example is the inability of the jaw to open fully.
MALOCCLUSION	A bad bite caused by the upper and lower teeth not fitting together properly.
MANDIBLE	The lower jaw, which forms the lower portion of the mouth.
MAXILLARY	The upper jaw.

MOLARS	Large, broad, multi-cusped teeth at the back of the mouth.
MOUTH GUARD	A soft, fitted device which protects teeth against impact or injury.
NEOPLASM	Refers to oral cancer.
NITROUS OXIDE	A gas inhaled to reduce anxiety in dental patients. Also called "laughing gas."
OCCLUSAL	Refers to the biting surface of the posterior teeth.
OCCLUSAL TRAUMA	Occurs when excessive forces are placed on a normal dentition (such as grinding and clenching of teeth). If left uncontrolled, may result in excessive wear or breaking teeth, in addition to attachment and bone loss.
OCCLUSION	Refers to the contact between maxillary and mandibular teeth in all mandibular positions and movement.
OPERATORY	A dental treatment room.
PERIAPICAL ABSCESS	Infection of the pulp of the tooth and tissues surrounding the base of the tooth.
PERIAPICAL X-RAYS	An x-ray that shows a tooth's crown, root, and surrounding bone structure.
PERIODONTAL	Of or pertaining to the tissue and bone that support teeth.
PERIODONTAL ABSCESS	Acute infection of the gingival tissues surrounding an individual tooth. Typically involves bone loss, pain, bleeding, severe redness, and swelling of the affected area.
PERIODONTAL DISEASE	Occurs when bacteria reside in the periodontal pocket, which can lead to tissue destruction. The pocket increases in depth and the tissue loses its ability to support the tooth in the alveolar bone.
PERIODONTAL LIGAMENT	The fibers which suspend the tooth in the bony socket. The periodontal ligament is attached at one end to the cementum and at the other end to the alveolar bone.

PERIODONTAL PROBE	An instrument used to measure pocket depth.
PERIODONTITIS	A form of periodontal disease affecting adults and resulting in destruction of alveolar bone.
PERMANENT TEETH	The adult teeth, usually 32 in number.
PLAQUE	A soft deposit of bacteria that grows on the teeth. When plaque hardens (calcifies) it is called "tartar."
PORCELAIN	A hard, tooth-colored substance used to make artificial crowns, especially in highly visible parts of the mouth where a natural appearance is important.
POSTERIOR TEETH	The premolar and molar teeth. The posterior teeth are those used for grinding food.
PROPHYLAXIS	A preventive dental office procedure involving tooth cleaning and polishing.
PULP	The living part of the tooth, located inside the dentin. Contains the nerve tissue and blood vessels which supply nutrients to the tooth.
RADIOGRAPHIC	Refers to to x-rays.
REMINERALIZATION	Replacement of the tooth's minerals into a demineralized area of the enamel.
RESISTANT BACTERIA	Bacteria which have developed resistance to typical modes of periodontal therapy.
RESTORATIONS	Any replacement for lost tooth structure or teeth (e.g., bridges, fillings, crowns, and implants).
SEALANTS	A plastic liquid which is placed on the top surfaces of posterior teeth. Used to prevent caries (tooth decay). The sealant hardens into place, forming a smooth surface that is easily cleaned with a toothbrush.
SUBGINGIVAL	The area below the gum line.

SULCUS	The moat-like space between the free gingival and the tooth. Has a depth of one to three millimeters.
SUPRAGINGIVAL	The area above the gingival margin.
TEETHING	Baby teeth pushing through gums.
TEMPOROMANDIBULAR	The area forming the joint.
JOINT	The "hinge" between the mandible and the skull.
THIRD MOLAR	The molar farthest back in the mouth. The last permanent tooth to erupt. Also called a "wisdom tooth."
TOPICAL	Refers to something applied directly to an infected area for treatment.
TOPICAL ANESTHETIC	A medication applied by spraying or swabbing the gum surface to lessen the pain of an oral injection.
TOPICAL FLUORIDE	A solution or gel containing fluoride which is applied to the outer surfaces of the teeth.
TOXICITY	Refers to the human safety level of a product or an ingredient.
ULTRASONIC	Conversion of high frequency electrical current into mechanical vibrations.
ULTRASONIC SCALER	A technology that uses ultrasonics to knock calculus, plaque, and endotoxins off of teeth.
VENEER	A cosmetic facing which adheres to the outer surface of a tooth. Also known as a "laminate."
XEROSTOMIA	A condition caused by the inadequate production of saliva by the salivary glands. Also called "dry mouth."

How To Order This Book

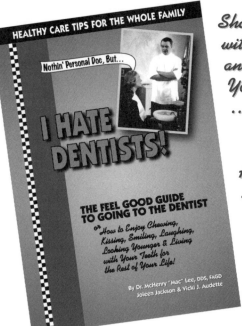

Share this book
with your friends
and dental patients.
You can order one book
... or many.

Ask about our
volume discounts.

1. **Call IHD Publishing**
   1-800-746-5486 (USA)
   1-254-547-9373 (outside USA)
   between the hours of
   8:00 a.m. and 5:00 p.m.

2. **Visit our Web site**
   http://www.ihatedentists.com

3. **Visit booksellers' Web sites.**
   Order the book 24 hours a day at:
   amazon.com or
   barnesandnoble.com

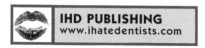

IHD PUBLISHING
www.ihatedentists.com

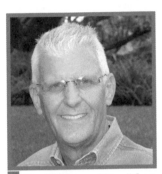

Dr. McHenry "Mac" Lee

Dr. Mac Lee is a third generation dentist, following in the professional footsteps of his father and grandfather, practicing at the Lee Dental Clinic- in Edna, Texas since 1910. Dr. Lee is a 1972 graduate of Baylor College of Dentistry in Dallas. He is a Fellow of the Academy of General Dentistry and a member of the American Dental Association. Since 1980, he has been teaching thousands of dentists and dental teams across America, Canada and Australia on how to have a consumer friendly dental practice. He co-authored *Nothin Personal Doc, But I Hate Dentists!* a dental consumer book that is making a difference in dentistry. Dr. Lee also developed ORA5 Antibacterial, used to treat canker sores in the mouth. Dr. Lee and his wife of 30+ years have three grown children.

Contact Dr. Lee at maclee@ihatedentists.com

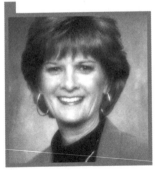

Joleen Jackson

Joleen Jackson has worn many hats during her 20-year career in dentistry. She has worked as a dental assistant, dental office administrator and a dental seminar presenter. She is the founder of a popular national dental newsletter, The Scoop. In 1980, Joleen became vice president of McHenry Laboratories. She is in charge of the marketing and sales division of ORA5®. Joleen assisted Dr. Lee with his nationally recognized seminars on gum disease. She works as an independent consultant to dentists and has trained dental team members across the United States and Canada. Through this experience, Joleen has studied hundreds of dental offices. In the last three years, she expanded her role as a speaker and trainer for dental teams to include a focus on the consumer to provide them with the information they need to make healthy dental decisions. She currently consults with dental teams, serving as an information liaison between dental professionals and their patients. Joleen has three daughters, and several grandchildren.

Contact Joleen Jackson at joleenjackson@ihatedentists.com

*V*icki Audette's media experience includes 20 years as a consumer reporter and TV producer in Minneapolis, Minnesota. Vicki is the author of several publications including *Dress Better for Less* and two consumer guidebooks. She understands that consumers want honest, straightforward information told in an informal, fun, understandable format.

She has appeared on the *Oprah Winfrey Show* several times, the Lifetime Cable Network, the *700 Club,* and numerous other radio and television shows in the United States. Vicki's consumer advice for finding quality goods and services has been featured in national magazines including *Family Circle, Gentleman's Quarterly,* and *Redbook.* She has also been featured in the major newspapers of cities such as Chicago, Los Angeles, Detroit, San Francisco, St. Paul, and Minneapolis.

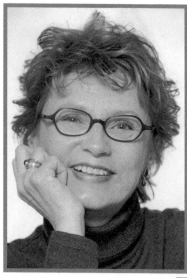

Vicki Audette

Ten years ago, Vicki moved to the Texas Hill Country to explore new frontiers and write the great American novel. But until her dream is fulfilled, she is focusing her consumer reporting talents on the dental profession.